DEMONSTRATING YOUR COMPETENCE 2: WOMEN'S HEALTH

Ruth Chambers
Gill Wakley
and
Julian Jenkins

RADCLIFFE MEDICAL PRESS
Oxford • San Francisco

Radcliffe Medical Press Ltd
18 Marcham Road
Abingdon
Oxon OX14 1AA
United Kingdom

www.radcliffe-oxford.com
The Radcliffe Medical Press electronic catalogue and online ordering facility.
Direct sales to anywhere in the world.

British Library Cataloguing in Publication Data

A catalogue record for this book is available from the British Library.

ISBN 1 85775 842 0

Typeset by Advance Typesetting Ltd, Oxfordshire
Printed and bound by TJ International Ltd, Padstow, Cornwall

Contents

Preface

The General Medical Council has asked doctors to start thinking now about how they will collect and keep the information that will show that they should continue to hold a licence to practise as doctors from 2005 onwards. The onus will be on individual doctors to show that they are up to date and fit to practise medicine throughout their careers. It will be doctors who decide for themselves the nature of the information they collect and retain that best reflects their roles and responsibilities in their everyday work.

This book is one of a series that will guide you as a general practitioner (GP) through the process, giving you examples and ideas as to how to document your learning, competence, performance or standards of service delivery. Chapter 1 explains the link between your personal development plans, local appraisal and the revalidation of your medical registration. Learning and service improvements that are integral to your personal development plan are central to the evidence you include in your appraisal and revalidation portfolio.

The stages of the evidence cycle that we suggest are built upon the under-pinning publication: Chambers R, Wakley G, Field S and Ellis S (2003) *Appraisal for the Apprehensive*. Radcliffe Medical Press, Oxford.

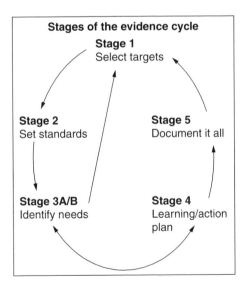

Stage 1 is about setting targets or aspirations for good practice. Many of the aspirations we suggest are taken from *Good Medical Practice*[1] or its sister publication, *Good Medical Practice for General Practitioners*.[2] Stage 2 encourages you, as a doctor, to set standards for the outcomes of what you plan to learn more about, or outcomes relating to you providing a good service in your practice.

Chapter 2 describes a variety of methods to help you to address Stage 3 of the cycle of evidence, to find out what it is you need to learn about or what gaps there are in the way you deliver care as an individual GP or as a team. This chapter includes a wide variety of methods doctors might use in their everyday work to identify and document these needs. One of the drivers for the introduction of appraisal and revalidation has been to reassure the public and others of doctors' continuing fitness to practise. So it makes sense that we have emphasised the importance of obtaining feedback from patients in this chapter in relation to identifying your learning and service development needs.

Best practice in addressing the giving of informed consent by patients, maintaining confidentiality of patient information and organising responsive complaints processes are all common components of good quality healthcare. Chapter 3 covers these aspects in depth and provides the first example of cycles of evidence for you to consider adopting or adapting for your own circum-stances. The focus of each cycle of evidence is on one of the 'headings' from *Good Medical Practice*[1] or the standard appraisal format.

The rest of the book consists of seven clinically based chapters that span key topics in women's health. The first part of each chapter covers key issues that are likely to crop up in typical consultations for each clinical field. The second part of each chapter gives examples of cycles of evidence in a similar format to those in Chapter 3.

Overall, you will probably want to choose three or four cycles of evidence each year. You might choose one or two from Chapter 3 and the rest from clinical areas such as those covered by Chapters 4 to 10. You might like this way of learning and service development so much that you build up a bigger bank of evidence, taking one cycle from each chapter in the same year. What-ever your approach, you will want to keep your cycles of evidence as short and simple as possible, so that the documentation itself is a by-product of the learning and action plans you undertake to improve the service you provide, and does not dominate your time and effort at work.

Other books in the series are based on the same format of the five stages in the cycle of evidence. Book 1 helps doctors and other health professionals to demonstrate that they are competent teachers or trainers, and Books 3, 4 and 5 set out key information and examples of evidence for a wide variety of clinical areas for GPs and other doctors.

This approach and style of learning will take a bit of getting used to for doctors. Until now, they have not had to prove that they are fit to practise unless the General Medical Council has investigated them for a significant reason such as a complaint or error. Until recently, most doctors did not evaluate what they learnt or whether they applied it in practice. They did not protect time for learning and reflection among their everyday responsibilities, or target their time and effort on priority topics. Times are changing, and with the introduction of personal development plans and appraisal GPs are realising that they must take a more professional approach to learning, and document their standards of competence, performance and service delivery. This book helps them to do just that.

Please note that resources to support this book are provided at <u>http://health.mattersonline.net</u>.

References

1 General Medical Council (2001) *Good Medical Practice*. General Medical Council, London.

2 Royal College of General Practitioners/General Practitioners' Committee (2002) *Good Medical Practice for General Practitioners*. Royal College of General Practitioners, London.

About the authors

Ruth Chambers has been a GP for more than 20 years and is currently the Head of the Stoke-on-Trent Teaching Primary Care Trust programme and Professor of Primary Care Development at Staffordshire University. Ruth has worked with the Royal College of General Practitioners to enable GPs to gather evidence about their learning and standards of practice while striving to be excellent GPs. Ruth has co-authored a series of books with Gill designed to help readers draw up their own personal development plans or workplace learning plans around key clinical topics.

Gill Wakley started in general practice but transferred to community medicine shortly afterwards and then into public health. A desire for increased contact with patients caused a move back into general practice. She has been heavily involved in learning and teaching throughout her career. She was in a training general practice, became an instructing doctor and a regional assessor in family planning, and was until recently a senior clinical lecturer with the Primary Care Department at Keele University. Like Ruth, she has run all types of educational initiatives and activities. A visiting professor at Staffordshire University, she now works as a freelance GP, writer and lecturer.

Julian Jenkins has had a longstanding involvement in postgraduate education and many initiatives including novel applications of learning technology. He is a consultant senior lecturer and the clinical director of the Centre for Reproductive Medicine at the University of Bristol (www.ReproMED.co.uk). He is the course director of an innovative MSc course in reproduction and development delivered principally over the Internet (www.ReD-MSc.org.uk) and the chairman of the Obstetrics and Gynaecology education subcommittee for the South West Region (www.swot.org.uk). For many years, he has been involved with the development of evidence-based medicine as a member of the Royal College of Obstetricians and Gynaecologists' Guidelines and Audit Committee and the Menstrual Disorder and Infertility Panel of the Cochrane Collaboration.

1

Making the link: personal development plans, appraisal and revalidation

The nexus of personal development plans, appraisal and revalidation

Learning involves many steps. It includes the acquisition of information, its retention, the ability to retrieve the information when needed and how to use that information for best practice. Demonstrating your learning involves being able to show the steps you have taken. Learning should be lifelong and encompass continuing professional development.

Continuing professional development (CPD) takes time. It makes sense to utilise the time spent by overlapping learning to meet your personal and professional needs, with that required for the performance of your role in the health service.

Many doctors have drawn up a personal development plan (PDP) that is agreed with their local CPD or college tutor. Some doctors have constructed their PDP in a systematic way and identified the priorities within it, or gathered evidence to demonstrate that what they learnt about was subsequently applied in practice. Tutors do not have a uniform approach to the style and relevance of a doctor's PDP. Some are content that a plan has been drawn up, while others encourage the doctor to develop a systematic approach to identifying and addressing their learning and service needs, in order of importance or urgency.[1]

The new emphasis on doctors' accountability to the public has given the PDP a higher profile and shown that it may be used in other ways. The medical education establishment and NHS management argue about the balance between its alternative uses. The educationalists view a PDP as a tool to encourage doctors to plan their own learning activities. The management view is of a tool allowing quality assurance of the doctor's performance. Doctors, striving to improve the quality of the care that they deliver to patients, want to use a PDP to guide them on their way, perhaps towards postgraduate awards of universities or the quality awards of the Royal College of General Practitioners

(RCGP). These quality awards are built around the standards of excellence to which a general practitioner (GP) should aspire, as described in the publication, *Good Medical Practice for General Practitioners.*[2]

Your personal development plan

Your PDP will be an integral part of your future appraisal and revalidation portfolio to demonstrate your fitness to practise as a doctor.

Your initial plan should:

- identify your gaps or weaknesses in knowledge, skills or attitudes
- specify topics for learning as a result of changes: in your role, responsibilities, the organisation in which you work
- link into the learning needs of others in your workplace or team of colleagues
- tie in with the service development priorities of your practice, the primary care organisation (PCO) or the NHS as a whole
- describe how you identified your learning needs
- set your learning needs and associated goals in order of importance and urgency
- justify your selection of learning goals
- describe how you will achieve your goals and over what time period
- describe how you will evaluate learning outcomes.

Each year you will continue or revise your PDP. It should demonstrate how you carried out your learning and evaluation plans, show that you have learnt what you set out to do (or why it was modified) and how you applied your new learning in practice. In addition, you will find that you have new priorities and fresh learning needs as circumstances change.

The main task is to capture what you have learnt, in a way that suits you. Then you can look back at what you have done and:

- reflect on it later, to decide to learn more, or to make changes as a result, and identify further needs
- demonstrate to others that you are fit to practise or work through:
  - what you have done
  - what you have learnt
  - what changes you have made as a result
  - the standards of work you have achieved and are maintaining
  - how you monitor your performance at work
- use it to show how your personal learning fits in with the requirements of your practice or the NHS, and other people's personal and professional development plans.

Organise all the evidence of your learning into a continuing professional development portfolio of some sort. It is up to you how you keep this record of your learning. Examples are:

- *an ongoing learning journal* in which you draw up and describe your plan, record how you determined your needs and prioritised them, report why you attended particular educational meetings or courses and what you got out of them as well as the continuing cycle of review, making changes and evaluating them
- *an A4 file* with lots of plastic sleeves into which you build up a systematic record of your educational activities in line with your plan
- *a box*: chuck in everything to do with your learning plan as you do it and sort it out into a sensible order every few months with a good review once a year.

The context of appraisal and revalidation

Appraisal and revalidation are based on the same sources of information – presented in the same structure as the headings set out in the General Medical Council (GMC) guidance in *Good Medical Practice*.[3] The two processes perform different functions. Whereas revalidation involves an assessment against a standard of fitness to practise medicine, appraisal is concerned with the doctor's professional development within his or her working environment and the needs of the organisation for which the doctor works.

Appraisal is a formative and developmental process that is being introduced by the Departments of Health for all GPs and hospital consultants working in the NHS across the UK. While the details of the appraisal system vary for consultants and GPs and for each of the countries, the educational principles remain the same. The aims of the appraisal system are to give doctors an opportunity to discuss and receive regular feedback on their previous and continuing performance and identify education and development needs.

The drive to introduce formal appraisals came initially as part of the programme to introduce clinical governance across the NHS as laid out in the 1998 consultation document *A First Class Service*.[4] Momentum was gained with the publication of *Supporting Doctors, Protecting Patients* (1999) in England which outlined a set of proposals to help prevent doctors from developing problems.[5] Appraisal was at the heart of the proposals as:

a positive process to give someone feedback on their performance, to chart their continuing progress and to identify development needs. It is a forward looking process essential for the developmental and educational planning needs of an individual. *Assessment* is the process of measuring progress against agreed criteria ... It is not the primary aim of appraisal to scrutinise doctors to see if they are performing poorly but rather to help them consolidate and improve on good performance aiming towards excellence.[5]

The document went on to suggest that appraisal should be made comprehensive and compulsory for doctors working in the NHS and form part of a future revalidation system.

In addition, appraisal should also address other areas of particular importance to the individual doctor. A standardised approach has been developed which utilises approved documentation. This should ensure that information from a variety of NHS employers is recorded consistently. The format of the paperwork is slightly different for consultants and GPs.

Appraisal must be a positive, formative and developmental process to support high quality patient care and improve clinical standards. Appraisal is different from, but linked to, revalidation.[6] Revalidation is the process whereby doctors will be regularly required to demonstrate that they are fit to practise. Appraisal feeds into this by contributing to the information that a doctor supplies for the revalidation process. Appraisal will provide a regular structured recording system for documenting progress towards revalidation and identifying needs as part of the doctor's PDP. Both the NHS appraisal and the revalidation structures are based on the same seven headings set out in the GMC's guidance *Good Medical Practice*.[3] The GMC claims, therefore, that 'five satisfactory appraisals equals revalidation'.[6] The GMC has also pledged that doctors not taking part in appraisal will be able to provide their own information for revalidation, providing this evidence meets the same criteria as in *Good Medical Practice*.[3]

Appraisal is, however, a two-way process. Not only time, but also resources will be needed to make appraisal systems successful. In addition, appraisal will identify issues that will require extra investment by the NHS in the educational and organisational infrastructure.

Appraisal and revalidation processes are being increasingly integrated. The PDP is a central part of the appraisal documentation, which will in turn be included in the portfolio of information available for revalidation. It seems that the evolution will continue so that revalidation is met by supporting the appraisal documentation with additional documents about clinical governance activity and CPD. These supporting documents will be a mix of subjective and objective information that will include doctors' self-assessment of their performance, and other work-based assessment.

The revalidation and appraisal processes need to be quality assured to be able to demonstrate that they can protect the public from poor or underperforming doctors. Such quality assurance will relate to the appraisers, their training and support, as well as systems to examine the quality of evidence in the documentation relating to a doctor's performance and outcomes of their

PDP. You should regard your PDP and supporting documentation as central to the way in which you can show, to anyone who requires you to do so, that your performance as a doctor is acceptable and that you are trying to improve, or striving for excellence.

Demonstrating the standards of your practice

The GMC sets out standards that must be met as part of the duties and responsibilities of doctors in the booklet *Good Medical Practice*.[3] Doctors must be able to meet these standards with a record of their own performance in their revalidation portfolio if they want to retain a licence to practise. The nine key headings of expected standards of practice for all GPs working in England are shown in Box 1.1.

Box 1.1: Key headings of expected standards of practice for GPs working in England

1 *Good professional practice.* This relates to clinical care, keeping records (including writing reports and keeping colleagues informed), access and availability, treatment in emergencies and making effective use of resources.

2 *Maintaining good medical practice.* This includes keeping up to date and maintaining your performance.

3 *Relationships with patients.* This encompasses providing information about your services, maintaining trust, avoiding discrimination and prejudice against patients, relating well to patients and apologising if things go wrong.

4 *Working with colleagues.* This relates to working with colleagues, working in teams, referring patients and accepting posts.

5 *Teaching and training, appraising and assessing.* You may be in a position to teach or train colleagues or students, and appraise or assess peers, employees or students.

6 *Probity* includes providing true information about your services, honesty in financial and commercial dealings, and providing references.

7 *Health* can include how you overcome or compensate for health problems in yourself, or help with or address health problems in other doctors.

8 *Research.* Conducting research in an ethical manner.

9 *Management.* The section on management concerns any responsibility GPs have for management outside the practice. GPs might wish to include management responsibilities that cross the interface between their practice and primary care organisation (PCO).

The appraisal paperwork for GPs working in England, Scotland, Wales and Northern Ireland has been individualised by each country. The English version, for example, includes two extra sections to those of hospital consultants, management and research. The Scottish version focuses on core categories in preparation for revalidation of prescribing, referrals and peer review, clinical audit, significant event analysis and communication skills, summary of any complaints and other feedback.

The stages of the evidence cycle for demonstrating your standards of practice or competence and any necessary improvements are given in Figure 1.1. The stages of the evidence cycle are common to all the various areas of expertise considered in this book and will be followed in each chapter.

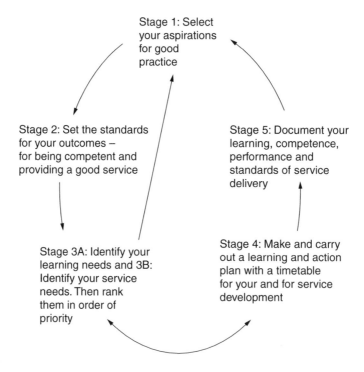

Figure 1.1:   Stages of the evidence cycle.

Although the five stages are shown in sequence here, in practice you would expect to move backwards and forwards from stage to stage, because of new information or a modification of your earlier ideas. New information might accrue when research is published which affects your clinical behaviour or standards, or a critical incident or patient complaint might occur which causes you and others to think anew about your standards or the way that services are delivered. The arrows in Figure 1.1 show that you might reset your target or aspirations for good practice, having undertaken exercises to identify what you need to learn or determine whether there are gaps in service delivery and, if so, what they are.

We suggest that you demonstrate your competence in focused areas of your day-to-day work by completing several cycles of evidence drawn from a variety of clinical or other areas each year, with at least one cycle of evidence from each of the main headings of *Good Medical Practice* over a five year cycle.[3] By demonstrating your standards of practice around the main sections of *Good Medical Practice*, you will document your competence and performance for your revalidation portfolio in the same format as that required for your appraisal paperwork.

As you start to collate information about this five stage cycle, discuss any problems about the standards of care or services you are looking at, with colleagues, experts in this area, tutors, etc. You want to develop a wide range and depth of evidence so that you can show that you are competent in your day-to-day general work as well as for any special areas of expertise.

Professional competence is the first area of concern in *Good Medical Practice*.[3] You should be able to demonstrate that you can maintain a satisfactory standard of clinical care most of the time in your everyday work. Some of the time you will be brilliant, of course! Celebrate those moments. On other occasions, you or others will be critical of your performance and feel that you could have done much better. Reflect on those episodes to learn from them.

Stage 1: Select your aspirations for good practice

By adopting or adapting descriptions of what an 'excellent' GP should be aiming for, you are defining the standards of practice for which all doctors should be aiming. The medical Royal Colleges have interpreted *Good Medical Practice* in various ways for the specialities of their own members.[3] For example, *Good Medical Practice for General Practitioners* describes the standards of practice that should be achieved by 'excellent' or 'unacceptable' GPs. Their definition of excellence is being 'consistently good'.[2]

This consistency is a critical factor in considering competence and performance too (*see* page 15). The documents that you collect in your evidence cycles must reflect consistency over time and in different circumstances, for example with various types of patients or your practice at different times of day. This will show that you have not only performed well on one occasion or for one type of baseline assessment, but also sustained your performance over time and under different conditions.

Stage 2: Set the standards for your outcomes – for being competent and providing a good service

Outcomes might include:

- the way that learning is applied
- a learnt skill
- a protocol
- a strategy that is implemented
- meeting recommended standards.

The level at which you should be performing depends on your particular field of expertise. GPs are good at seeing the wider picture, while specialists tend to be expert in a narrow area, so that the level of competence expected for a clinical area will vary depending on the doctor's role and responsibilities. You would not, for example, expect orthopaedic specialists to be competent at managing cardiac failure (although some of them may be), but you would expect GPs to be able to manage all but the most complicated situations involving cardiac failure. You would expect both the orthopaedic specialist and the GP to recognise the limits of their competence and to refer to someone with more expertise when necessary.

Other standards include using resources effectively and the record keeping that is an essential tool in clinical care. As a health professional, you need to be accessible and available so that you can provide your services, and make suitable arrangements for handing over care to others. You must provide care in an emergency.

You could incorporate into your standards or outcomes those components specified by universities at a national level as part of their Masters' Frameworks for their postgraduate awards. The Masters' Frameworks consist of eight components that shape the individual postgraduate award programme outcomes and the learning outcomes of the individual modules for the postgraduate awards. The eight components are shown in Box 1.2. You could set out your CPD work in the portfolio you are assembling for revalidation and your annual appraisals in this format. This would help you to document your professional development to date in a form that can be readily 'accredited for prior experiential learning' (APEL) by universities (contact your local universities if you want more information about this process). You might then be given credits for learning against an intended postgraduate award. It would save you from duplicating work as well as speeding your progress through the award.

If you have information or data about your practice showing that it was substandard or that you were not competent, you might choose to exclude that from your portfolio. However, you will be able to show that you have learnt more by reviewing mistakes or negative episodes. It is better to include everything

---

Box 1.2:   The eight components of the Masters' Frameworks for postgraduate awards

1   Analysis
2   Problem solving
3   Knowledge and understanding
4   Reflection
5   Communication
6   Learning
7   Application
8   Enquiry

---

of relevance, then go on to demonstrate how you addressed the gaps in your performance and made sustained improvements. You will need to protect the confidentiality of patients and colleagues as necessary when you collect data. The GMC will be seeing the contents of your revalidation portfolio if your submission is one of those sampled. You will probably also submit or share the documentation for appraisal and maybe use it for reviews with colleagues or the primary care organisation.

Stage 3: Identify your learning and service needs in your practice or primary care organisation and rank them in order of priority[1]

The type and depth of documentation you need to gather will encompass:

• the context in which you work
• your knowledge and skills in relation to any particular role or responsibility of your current post.

The extent of expertise you should possess will depend on your level of responsibility for a particular function or task. You may be personally responsible for that function or task, or you may contribute or delegate responsibility for it. Your learning needs should take into account your aspirations for the future too – personal or career development for you, or improvements in the way you deliver care in your practice. Look at Chapter 2 for more ideas on how you will identify your learning or service development needs.

Group and summarise your service development needs from the exercises you have carried out. Grade them according to the priority you set. You may put one at a higher priority because it fits in with service development needs established in the business plan of the trust or practice, or put another lower because it does not fit in with other activities that your organisation has in their current development plan for the next 12 months. If you have identified a service development need by several different methods of assessment or with several different patient groups or clinical conditions, then it will have a higher priority than something only identified once. Notify the service development needs you have identified to those responsible for agreeing and implementing the development plans of the trust and/or practice.

Look back at your aspirations and standards set out in Stages 1 and 2. Match your learning or service development needs with one or more of these standards, or others that you have set yourself.

Stage 4: Make and carry out a learning and action plan with a timetable for your personal and service development

If you have not identified any learning needs for yourself or the service as a whole, you should omit Stage 4 and tidy up the presentation of your evidence for inclusion in your portfolio as at the end of Stage 5.

Think about whether:

* you have defined your learning objectives – what you need to learn to be able to attain the standards and outcomes you have described in Stage 2
* you can justify spending time and effort on the topics you prioritised in Stage 3. Is the topic important enough to your work, the NHS as a whole or patient safety? Does the clinical or non-clinical event occur sufficiently often to warrant the time spent?
* the time and resources for learning about that topic or making the associated changes to service delivery are available. Check that you are not trying to do too much too quickly, or you will become discouraged
* learning about that topic will make a difference to the care you or others can provide for patients
* and how one topic fits in with other topics you have identified to learn more about. Have you achieved a good balance across your areas of work or between your personal aspirations and the basic requirements of the service?

Decide on what method of learning is most appropriate for your task or role or the standards you are expecting to attain or sustain. You may have already identified your preferred learning style – but read up on this elsewhere if you are unsure.[7]

Describe how you will carry out your learning tasks and what you will do by a specified time. State how your learning will be applied and how and when it will be evaluated. Build in some staging posts so that you do not suddenly get to the end of 12 months and discover that you have only done half of your plan.

Your action plan should also include your role in remedying any gaps in service delivery that you identified in Stage 3 and that are within the remit of your responsibility.

Stage 5: Document your learning, competence, performance and standards of service delivery

You might choose to document that you have attained your defined outcomes by repeating the learning needs assessment that you started with. You could record your increased confidence and competence in dealing with situations that you previously avoided or performed inadequately.

You might incorporate your assessment of what has been gained in a study of another area that overlaps.

Preparing your portfolio[8-10]

Use your portfolio of evidence of what you have learnt and your standards of practice to:

- identify significant experiences to serve as important sources of learning
- reflect on the learning that arose from those experiences
- demonstrate learning in practice
- analyse and identify further learning needs and ways in which these needs can be met.

Your documentation might include all sorts of things, not just formal audits – although they make a good start. It might include reports of educational activities attended, statements of your roles and responsibilities, copies of publications you have read and critically appraised, and reports of your work. You could incorporate observations by others, evaluations of you observing other colleagues and how their practice differs from yours, descriptions of self-improvements, a video of typical activity, materials that demonstrate your skills to others, products of your input or learning – a new protocol for example. Box 1.3 gives a list of material you might include in your portfolio.

Once you are preparing to submit the portfolio for a discussion with a colleague (for example, at an appraisal) or assessment (for example, for a university postgraduate award or revalidation) write a self-assessment of your previous action plan. You might integrate your self-assessment into your PDP

Box 1.3:   Possible contents of a portfolio
- Workload logs
- Case descriptions
- Videos
- Audiotapes
- Patient satisfaction surveys
- Research surveys
- Report of change or innovation
- Commentaries on published literature or books
- Records of critical incidents and learning points
- Notes from formal teaching sessions with reference to clinical work or other evidence

---

to show what you have achieved and what gaps you have still to address. Decide where you are now and where you want to be in one, three or five years' time. Select items from your portfolio for inclusion for each part of the documentation – you might have one compartment of your portfolio per speciality topic or section heading from *Good Medical Practice*.[3]

Make sure all references are included and the documentation in your portfolio is as accurate and complete as possible. Organise how you have shown your learning steps and your standards of practice so that it is indexed and cross-referenced to the relevant sections of the paperwork. Discuss the contents of your portfolio with a colleague or a mentor to gain other people's perspectives of your work and look for blind-spots.

Include evidence of your competence as a GP with a special interest (GPwSI)

You may have a particular expertise or special interest in a clinical field or non-clinical area such as management, teaching or research. It may be that you have a lead role or responsibility in your practice for chronic disease management of clinical conditions such as diabetes, asthma, mental health or coronary heart disease. Or you may be employed by a primary care organisation or hospital trust as a GPwSI to:

- lead in the development of services
- deliver a procedure-based service
- deliver an opinion-based service.

There is little consistency in extent of training or qualifications at present within or across the various GPwSI speciality areas.[11] Whatever your role or responsibility or expertise, your portfolio should include examples of evidence that show that you are competent, and that you have a consistently good performance in your speciality area. You may have parallel appraisals that you can include from your employer – for example, the university if you have a research or teaching post, or a hospital consultant if he or she supervises you in the clinical speciality.

When you gather evidence of your performance at work, try to document as many aspects of your work at one time as you can, so that for example an audit covers as many of the key headings from *Good Medical Practice* (*see* page 5) as possible.[3] When you are identifying what you need to learn, or gaps in service delivery, make sure that you involve patients and show how you interact with the team. This gives you evidence about 'relationships with patients' and 'working with colleagues' as well as the clinical area you are focusing on or auditing.

Link your cycles of evidence to service developments rewarded by the new General Medical Services (GMS) Contract or Personal Medical Services (PMS) arrangements

The areas within the quality framework will probably be the ones that you prioritise in your PDP when looking at your service development needs.[12] The four main components of the quality framework are all relevant to your personal and professional development. The clinical and organisational standards may be those which you are aiming for in Stage 2 of the evidence cycle (*see* Figure 1.1). Achieving the standards in the quality framework will follow on from the descriptions of an excellent GP (Stage 1). Identifying personal learning needs and service development needs, that is, the gaps between baseline and specified standards in the quality framework, is in Stage 3. Making and carrying out your personal learning plan and service improvements in line with patients' experience is in Stage 4. Producing the documentation that shows you have attained the clinical or organisational standards required for core or additional services and responded to patients' views is in Stage 5.

References

1 Wakley G, Chambers R and Field S (2000) *Continuing Professional Development in Primary Care.* Radcliffe Medical Press, Oxford.

2 Royal College of General Practitioners/General Practitioners' Committee (2002) *Good Medical Practice for General Practitioners.* Royal College of General Practitioners, London.

3 General Medical Council (2001) *Good Medical Practice.* General Medical Council, London.

4 Department of Health (1998) *A First Class Service.* Department of Health, London.

5 Department of Health (1999) *Supporting Doctors, Protecting Patients.* Department of Health, London.

6 General Medical Council (2003) *Licence to Practise and Revalidation for Doctors.* General Medical Council, London. www.revalidationuk.info.

7 Mohanna K, Wall D and Chambers R (2003) *Teaching Made Easy: a manual for health professionals* (2e). Radcliffe Medical Press, Oxford.

8 Royal College of General Practitioners (1993) *Portfolio-based Learning in General Practice.* Occasional Paper 63, Royal College of General Practitioners, London.

9 Challis M (1999) AMEE Medical education guide No 11 (revised): portfolio-based learning and assessment in medical education. *Medical Teacher.* **21(4)**: 370–86.

10 Chambers C, Wakley G, Field S and Ellis S (2003) *Appraisal for the Apprehensive.* Radcliffe Medical Press, Oxford.

11 www.gpwsi.org.

12 General Practitioners' Committee/The NHS Confederation (2003) *New GMS Contract. Investing in general practice.* General Practitioners' Committee, London.

2

Practical ways to identify your learning and service needs as part of the documentation of your competence and performance

Setting standards to show that you are competent

> Doctors 'must be committed to lifelong learning and be responsible for maintaining the medical knowledge and clinical and team skills necessary for the provision of quality care'.[1]

You could make a good start by describing your roles and responsibilities. This will help you to define what your competence should be now, or what competence you are hoping to attain (for instance as a GPwSI). Once you have your definition, you can recognise whether you have, or lack in some part, the necessary competence. If there are no accepted descriptions of competence in the area you are focusing on, then you will have to start from scratch. You might compile your description from national guidelines such as in the National Service Frameworks or health strategies. Usually you can find guidance about competency from specialist sources such as primary care associations for clinical topics or the various Royal Colleges. The Department of Health in England has worked with the Royal College of General Practitioners (RCGP) to describe the competency of GPs with special clinical interests in many clinical areas.[2]

A good definition of competence is someone who is 'able to perform the tasks and roles required to the expected standard'.[3]

You will need to describe the standards expected in the range of tasks and roles you undertake and reference the source of standard setting. If professionals, or their organisations, are the only people involved in setting those standards, consider whether you should amend or extend the standards, tasks or roles by considering other perspectives such as those of patients or the NHS as a whole.

There is a difference between being competent, and performing in a consistently competent manner. You need to be motivated to perform consistently well and enabled to do so with efficient systems and sufficient resources. You will require sufficient numbers of other competent doctors or staff and available infrastructure such as diagnostic and treatment resources.[4]

Choose methods in Stage 3 (*see* Chapter 1) to demonstrate your standards of performance and identify any learning needs that span different topic areas, to reduce duplication and maximise the usefulness of your learning. Collecting evidence of more than one aspect of your competence or performance cuts down the overall amount of work underpinning your PDP or included in your appraisal portfolio.

Use several methods to identify your learning needs and/or gaps in your service development or delivery, so that you validate the findings of one method by another. No one method will give you reliable information about the gaps in your knowledge, skills or attitudes or everyday service. Does what you think about your performance match with what others in the team or patients think of how you practise in your everyday work? It is particularly difficult to determine what it is you 'don't know you don't know' by yourself, yet it is vital that you identify and rectify those gaps. Other people may be able to tell you quite readily what you need to learn. Colleagues from different disciplines could usefully comment on any shortfalls in how your work interfaces with theirs.

Patients or people who don't use your services could tell you whether the way you operate or provide services is off-putting or inappropriate. There may be data about your performance or that of your practice that could point out those gaps in your knowledge or skills of which you were previously unaware.

Determine what it is that you 'don't know you don't know' by:

- asking patients, users and non-users of your service
- comparing your performance against best practice or that of peers
- comparing your performance against objectives in business plans or national directives
- asking colleagues from different disciplines about shortfalls in how your work interfaces with theirs.

Stage 3A: Identify your learning needs – how you can find out if you need to be better at doing your job

You may decide to use a few selected methods to gather baseline evidence of your performance, focused on your specific area of expertise. You may target other topics or areas at the same time that are relevant to the various sections of the GMC's booklet *Good Medical Practice*.[5] For this type of combined assessment, you might use several of the methods described in this chapter such as:

- constructive feedback from peers or patients
- 360° feedback
- self-assessment, or review by others, using a rating scale to assess your skills and attitudes
- comparison with protocols and guidelines for checking how well procedures are followed
- audit: various types and applications
- significant event audit
- eliciting patient views such as in satisfaction surveys
- a SWOT (strengths, weaknesses, opportunities and threats) or SCOT (strengths, challenges, opportunities and threats) analysis
- reading and reflecting
- educational review.

Several of these methods will also be useful for identifying service development needs – you can look at the gaps identified from both the personal and service perspectives at the same time using the same method.

Seek feedback

Find colleagues who will give you constructive feedback about your performance and practice. The golden rule for giving constructive feedback is to give positive praise of things that have been well done first. Sometimes colleagues launch straight in to criticise faults when asked for their views. The Pendleton model of giving feedback is widely used in the health setting (*see* Box 2.1).[6]

Box 2.1: The Pendleton model of giving feedback[6]

1 The 'learner' goes first and performs the activity.
2 Questions clarify any facts.
3 The 'learner' says what they thought was done well.
4 The 'teacher' says what they thought was done well.
5 The 'learner' says what could be improved upon.
6 The 'teacher' says what could be improved upon.
7 Both discuss ideas for improvements in a helpful and constructive manner.

360° feedback

This collects together perceptions from a number of different participants as shown in Figure 2.1.

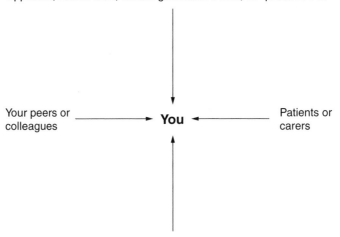

Figure 2.1:   360° feedback.

The wider the spread of people giving feedback, the more rounded the picture. Each individual gives a feedback questionnaire to at least three people in each of the groups above. An independent person then collects and collates the questionnaires and discusses the results with the individual. Computerised versions are available from commercial companies.[7] The main disadvantage of this method is that it can sometimes be spoilt by malicious comments against which individuals cannot readily defend themselves.

Self-assess or gain another person's perspective on your standard of practice or service delivery

You might describe any aspect of your practice as statements (A to G as in Box 2.2) about your competence or performance for you to self-assess, or others to give you feedback or comments by marking the extent to which they agree on the linear scales below. You could use the descriptions of an excellent GP in *Good Medical Practice for General Practitioners*[8] as we have done in relating statements in Box 2.2 to consultation skills. For instance, if statement A is: 'I consistently treat patients politely and with consideration', you could self-assess the extent to which you agree. Alternatively, you could ask colleagues or patients to fill in the assessment form. Objective feedback from external assessment is usually more reliable than your own self-assessment when you may have blind-spots about your own performance. As you become more confident in this method of reviewing your competence, you might emphasise how consistent you are in your application of good practice – so in the statements below we have sometimes included 'consistently', 'always' or 'usually'. You can set your own challenges. If you have a mentor or a 'buddy' in the practice with whom you learn, you might discuss and reflect on the completed marking grids with him or her.

Box 2.2: Marking grid: circle the number which represents your views or feelings about each statement – complete the grid on more than one occasion and compare results over time

A   I consistently treat patients politely and with consideration.

STRONGLY AGREE   to   STRONGLY DISAGREE

1------------------2------------------3------------------4------------------5------------------6

B   I am aware of how my personal beliefs could affect the care offered to the patient, and take care not to impose my own beliefs and values.

STRONGLY AGREE   to   STRONGLY DISAGREE

1------------------2------------------3------------------4------------------5------------------6

C   I always treat all patients equally and ensure that some groups are not favoured at the expense of others.

STRONGLY AGREE   to   STRONGLY DISAGREE

1------------------2------------------3------------------4------------------5------------------6

continued overleaf

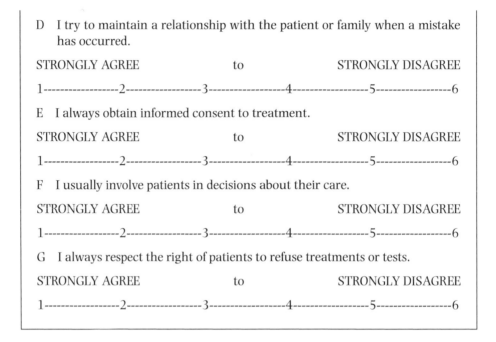

D   I try to maintain a relationship with the patient or family when a mistake has occurred.

STRONGLY AGREE   to   STRONGLY DISAGREE

1------------------2------------------3------------------4------------------5------------------6

E   I always obtain informed consent to treatment.

STRONGLY AGREE   to   STRONGLY DISAGREE

1------------------2------------------3------------------4------------------5------------------6

F   I usually involve patients in decisions about their care.

STRONGLY AGREE   to   STRONGLY DISAGREE

1------------------2------------------3------------------4------------------5------------------6

G   I always respect the right of patients to refuse treatments or tests.

STRONGLY AGREE   to   STRONGLY DISAGREE

1------------------2------------------3------------------4------------------5------------------6

Compare your performance against protocols or guidelines

Are you familiar with all the protocols or guidelines that are used by someone, somewhere in the practice? You might determine your learning needs and those of other practice team members by piling all the protocols or guidelines that exist in your practice in a big heap and rationalising them so that you have a common set across the practice. Working as a team you can compare your own knowledge and usual practice with others and with protocols or guidelines recommended by the National Institute for Clinical Excellence (NICE)[9] or National Service Frameworks or the Scottish Intercollegiate Guidelines Network (SIGN).[10]

Alternatively, you might compare your own practice against a protocol or guideline that is generally accepted at a national or local level. You could audit the standard of your practice to find out how often you adhere to such a protocol or guideline, and if you can justify why you deviate from the recommendations.

Audit

Audit is:

the method used by health professionals to assess, evaluate, and improve the care of patients in a systematic way, to enhance their health and quality of life.[11]

The five steps of the audit cycle are shown in Box 2.3.

Box 2.3: The five steps of the audit cycle

1 Describe the criteria and standards you are trying to achieve.
2 Measure your current performance of how well you are providing care or services in an objective way.
3 Compare your performance against criteria and standards.
4 Identify the need for change – to performance, adjustment of criteria or standards, resources, available data.
5 Make any required changes as necessary and re-audit later.

Performance or practice is often broken down for the purposes of audit into the three aspects of structure, process and outcome. Structural audits might concern resources such as equipment, premises, skills, people, etc. Process audits focus on what is done to the patient: for instance, clinical protocols and guidelines. Audits of outcomes consider the impact of care or services on the patient and might include patient satisfaction, health gains and effectiveness of care or services. You might look at aspects of quality of the structure, process and outcome of the delivery of any clinical field, focusing on access, equity of care between different groups in the population, efficiency, economy, effectiveness for individual patients, etc.[12]

Set standards for your performance, find out how you are doing, search to find out best practice, make the changes and then re-audit the care given to patients in the future with the same problem. Some variations on audit include:

- *Case note analysis.* This gives an insight into your current practice. It might be a retrospective review of a random selection of notes, or a prospective survey of consecutive patients with the same condition as they present to see you.
- *Peer review.* Compare an area of practice with other individual professionals or managers, or compare practice teams as a whole. An independent body might compare all practices in one area e.g. within a primary care organisation (PCO) so that like is compared with like. Feedback may be

arranged to protect participants' identities so that only the individual person or practice knows their own identity, the rest being anonymised, for example by giving each practice a number. Where there is mutual trust and an open learning culture, peer review does not need to be anonymised and everyone can learn together about making improvements in practice.

- *Criteria based audit*. This compares clinical practice with specific standards, guidelines or protocols. Re-audit of changes should demonstrate improvements in the quality of patient care.
- *External audit*. Prescribing advisers or managers in PCOs can supply information about indicators of performance for audit. Visits from external bodies such as the Commission for Healthcare Audit and Inspection (CHAI) expose the PCO or hospital trust in England and Wales to external audit.
- *Tracer criteria*. Assessing the quality of care of a 'tracer' condition may be used to represent the quality of care of other similar conditions or more complex problems. Tracer criteria should be easily defined and measured. For instance, if you were to audit the extent to which you reviewed repeat prescriptions, you might focus on a drug such as thyroxine and generalise from your audit results to your likely performance with other medications.

Significant event audit

Think of an incident where a patient or you experienced an adverse event. This might be an unexpected death, an unplanned pregnancy, an avoidable side-effect from prescribed medication, a violent attack on a member of staff, or an angry outburst in public by you or a work colleague. You can review the case and reflect on the sequence of events that led to that critical event occurring. It is likely that there were a multitude of factors leading up to that significant event. You should take the case to a multidisciplinary meeting to reflect and analyse what were the triggers, causes and consequences of the event. Complete the significant event audit cycle by planning what individuals, or the practice as a whole, might do to avoid a similar event happening in future. This might include undertaking further learning and/or making appropriate changes to the practice or your systems.

The steps of a significant event audit are shown in Box 2.4.

Box 2.4:   Steps of a significant event audit

- *Step 1*: Describe who was involved, what time of day, what the task/activity was, the context and any other relevant information.
- *Step 2*: Reflect on the effects of the event on the participants and the professionals involved.
- *Step 3*: Discuss the reasons for the event or situation arising with other colleagues, review case notes or other records.
- *Step 4*: Decide how you or others might have behaved differently. Describe your options for how the procedures at work might be changed to minimise or eliminate chances of the event recurring.
- *Step 5*: Plan changes that are needed, how they will be implemented, who will be responsible for what and when, what further training or resources are required. Then carry out the changes.
- *Step 6*: Re-audit later to see whether changes to procedures or new knowledge and skills are having the desired effects. Give feedback to the practice team.

An assessment by an external body

This is a traditional way of showing that you are competent by taking and passing an examination. It is a good way of testing recalled knowledge in a written or oral examination, or establishing how you behave in a clinical situation on the day of a practical examination, but not much good for measuring anything else. A summative examination (i.e. done at the end of a course of study) gives a measure of your learning up to that date.

You might undertake an objective test of your knowledge and skills. Examples are a computer-based test in the form of multiple-choice questions and patient management problems as in the RCGP's phased evaluation programme (PEP) CD ROMs (email pep@rcgp-scotland.org.uk) or the Apollo programme available from BMJ Publishing.[13] Various other organisations give multiple-choice questionnaires that you can complete on paper[14] or online[15] and record in your portfolio.

The RCGP's series of quality awards provide external assessment – Membership by Assessment of Performance, Fellowship by Assessment, Quality Team Development, etc. Trained assessors will give feedback to individual doctors or practice teams about their performance compared with set standards and their peers.

Elicit the views of patients

Part of meeting the criteria for relationships with patients in *Good Medical Practice*[5] might be to assess patients' satisfaction with:

* you
* your practice
* the local hospital's way of working
* other services available in your locality.

Avoid surveys where questions are relatively superficial or biased. A more specific enquiry should uncover particular elements of patients' dissatisfaction, which will be more useful if you are trying to identify your learning needs. Use a well-validated patient questionnaire instead of risking producing your own version with ambiguities and flaws such as the General Practice Assessment Questionnaire (GPAQ)[16] or the Doctors' Interpersonal Skills Questionnaire (DISQ).[17] Many doctors and practice teams have used these patient survey methods, providing a bank of data against which to compare your performance.

Other sources of feedback from patients might be obtained through suggestion boxes for patients to contribute comments, or the practice team recording all patients' suggestions and complaints however trivial, looking for patterns in the comments received.

There will be learning to be had from every complaint – even if the complaint does not have any substance, there should be something to learn about the shortfall in communication between you and the complainant.

The evolving of the 'expert patient programme' should mean that there is a pool of well-informed patients with chronic conditions who can contribute their insights into what you (or the service) need to learn from a patient's perspective.[18]

Strengths, weaknesses (or challenges), opportunities and threats (SWOT or SCOT) analysis

You can undertake a SWOT (or SCOT) analysis of your own performance or that of your practice team or practice organisation, working it out on your own, or with a workmate or mentor, or with a group of colleagues. Brainstorm the strengths, weaknesses (or challenges), opportunities and threats of your role or circumstances.

Strengths and weaknesses (or challenges) of your roles might relate to your clinical knowledge or skills, experience, expertise, decision making, communication skills, interprofessional relationships, political skills, timekeeping, organisational skills, teaching skills, or research skills. Strengths and weaknesses (or challenges) of the practice organisation might relate to most of these aspects as well as the way resources are allocated, overall efficiency and the degree to which the practice is patient-centred.

Opportunities might relate to your unexploited experience or potential strengths, expected changes in the NHS, or resources for which you might bid. For example, you might train for and set up a special interest post.

Threats will include factors and circumstances that prevent you from achieving your aims for personal, professional and practice development or service improvements. They might be to do with your health, turnover in the practice team, or time-limited investment by the PCO.

List the important factors in your SWOT (or SCOT) analysis in order of priority through discussion with colleagues and independent people from outside your practice. Draw up goals and a timed action plan for you or the practice team to follow.

Informal conversations – in the corridor, over coffee

You learn such a lot when chatting with colleagues at coffee time or over a meal and can become aware of your learning or service development needs at these times. This is when you realise that other people are doing things differently from you and if they seem to be doing it better and achieving more, you can challenge yourself to decide if this matter could be one of your blind-spots. Note down your thoughts before you forget them so that you can reflect on them later.

Online discussion groups may provide another source of informal exchanges with colleagues. If you find this difficult to start with, you might 'lurk', viewing the comments and views of other people until you feel confident enough to contribute. Record any observations that you find useful and reflect on how they might inform your own practice.

Observe your work environment and role

Observation could be informal and opportunistic, or more systematic, working through a structured checklist. One method of self-assessment might be to audiotape yourself at work dealing with patients (after obtaining patients' informed consent). Listen to the tape afterwards to appraise your communication and consultation skills – on your own or with a friend or colleague. If you have access to video equipment, you might use this instead.

Look at the equipment in your practice or your emergency bag. Do you know how to operate it properly? Assess yourself undertaking practical procedures or ask someone to watch you operate the equipment or undertaking the practical procedure and give you feedback about your performance.

Analyse the various roles and responsibilities of your current posts. Compare your level of expertise against national standards such as in the Knowledge and Skills Framework for England from the Department of Health or a job evaluation framework as part of the Agenda for Change initiative.[19,20] Determine if you can meet the requirements, or, if not, what deficiencies need to be made good.

You might combine one of the methods of identifying your learning needs already described such as an audit or SWOT analysis and apply it to 'observing your work environment or role', describing your relationship with other members of the multidisciplinary team for example, or reviewing how their roles and responsibilities interface with yours.

Reading and reflecting

When reading articles in respected journals, reflect on what the key messages mean for you in your situation. Note down topics about which you know little but that are relevant to your work, and calculate if you have further learning needs not met by the article you are reading. If the article is relevant to your practice, record what changes you will make and how you will make the changes. Record how you will impart your new knowledge to others in your practice.

Educational review

You might find a buddy or work colleague, CPD tutor, or a clinical tutor or clinical supervisor with whom you can have an informal or formal discussion about your performance, job situation and learning needs. You might draw up a learning contract as a result with a timed plan of action.

Stage 3B: Identify your service needs – how you can find out if there are gaps in services or how you deliver care

Now focus your attention on the needs of your practice or the PCO. The standards of service delivery should be those that allow you to practise as a competent clinician. You may be competent but be unable to perform or practise to a competent level if the resources available to you are inadequate, or other colleagues have insufficient knowledge or skills to support you. You cannot be expected to take responsibility for ensuring that resources you need to be able to practise in a competent manner are available. However, as a professional you should play a significant role in collecting evidence to make a case for the need for essential resources to your GP colleagues, the practice manager, staff at the trust or PCO or whoever is appropriate.

Some of the methods you might use are described below and include:

- involving patients and the public in giving you feedback about the quality and quantity of your services
- monitoring access and availability to care
- undertaking a force-field analysis
- assessing risk
- evaluating the standards of care or services you provide
- comparing the systems in your practice with those required by legislation
- considering your patient population's health needs
- reviewing teamwork
- assessing the quality of your services
- reflecting on whether you are providing cost-effective care and services.

Involve patients and the public in giving you feedback about the quality and quantity of your services

Patient and public involvement may occur at three levels:

1   for individual patients about their own care
2   for patients and the public about the range and quality of health services on offer
3   in planning and organising health service developments.

The phrase 'patient and public involvement' is used here to mean individual involvement as a user, patient or carer; or public involvement that includes the processes of consultation and participation.[21]

If a patient involvement or public consultation exercise is to be meaningful, it has to involve people who represent the section of the population that the exercise is about. You will have to set up systems to actively seek out and involve people from minority groups or those with sensory impairments such as blind and deaf people.

Before you start:

- define the purpose
- be realistic about the magnitude of the planned exercise
- select an appropriate method or several methods depending on the target population and your resources

- obtain the commitment of everyone who will be affected by the exercise
- frame the method in accordance with your perspective
- write the protocol.

You might hold focus groups, or set up a patient panel, or invite feedback and help from a patient participation group. You could interview patients selected either at random from the patient population or for their experience of a particular condition or circumstance.

Monitor access and availability to healthcare

Access and availability

You could look at waiting times to see a health professional by using:

- computerised appointment lists or paper and pen to record the time of arrival, the time of the appointment, the time seen
- the next available appointments which can easily be monitored by computer, or more painfully by manual searches of the appointment books.

Compare the results at intervals (a spreadsheet is a good way to do this). Do you or your staff have learning needs in relation to the use of technology, or new ways of redesigning the service you offer?

Referrals to other agencies and hospitals

You might audit and re-audit the time taken from the date the patient is seen to:

- the referral being sent (do you need more secretarial time?)
- the date the patient is seen by the other agency (could the patient be seen elsewhere quicker or do you need to liaise with other agencies over referrals?)
- the date the patient's needs have been met by investigation, diagnosis, treatment, provision of aid or support, etc. (can you influence how quickly these are completed?).

Identify any learning needs here. For instance, new methods of teamwork with a different mix of skills between doctors, nurses and non-clinically qualified assistants could provide extra services in the practice, or you, or a colleague, might retrain to become a GP with a special clinical interest.

Draw up a force-field analysis

This tool will help you to identify and focus down on the positive and negative forces in your work and to gain an overview of the weighting of these factors.

Draw a horizontal or vertical line in the middle of a sheet of paper. Label one side 'positive' and the other side 'negative'. Draw bars to represent individual positive drivers that motivate you on one side of the line, and factors that are demotivating on the other negative side of the line. The thickness and length of the bars should represent the extent of the influence; that is, a short, narrow bar will indicate that the positive or negative factor has a minor influence and a long, wide bar a major effect. *See* Box 2.5 for an example.

Box 2.5: Example of force-field analysis diagram. Satisfaction with current post as a health professional

Positive factors (driving forces)	Negative factors (restraining forces)
career aspirations	long hours of work
salary	demands from patients
autonomy	
satisfaction from caring	job insecurity
no uniform	oppressive hierarchy
opportunities for professional development	

Take an overview of the resulting force-field diagram and consider if you are content with things as they are, or can think of ways to boost the positive side and minimise the negative factors. You can do this part of the exercise on your own, with a peer or a small group in the practice, or with a mentor or someone from outside the practice. The exercise should help you to realise the extent to which a known influence in your life, or in the practice as a whole, is a positive or negative factor. Make a personal or organisational action plan to create the situations and opportunities to boost the positive factors in your life and minimise the bars on the negative side.

Assess risk

Risk assessment might entail evaluating the risks to the health or wellbeing or competence of yourself, staff and/or patients in your practice or workplace, and deciding on the action needed to minimise or eliminate those risks.[22]

- *A hazard*: something with the potential to cause harm.
- *A risk*: the likelihood of that potential to cause harm being realised.

There are five steps to risk assessment:

1   Look for and list the hazards.
2   Decide who might be harmed and how.
3   Evaluate the risks arising from the hazards and decide whether existing precautions are adequate or more should be done.
4   Record the findings.
5   Review your assessment from time to time and revise it if necessary.

You do not want to spend a lot of time and effort identifying risks or making changes if they do not matter much. When you have identified a risk, consider:

- is the risk large?
- does it happen often?
- is it a significant risk?

Risks may be prevented, avoided, minimised or managed where they cannot be eliminated. You, your colleagues and your staff may need to learn how to do this.

Record significant events where someone has experienced an adverse event or had a near miss – as part of you identifying your service development needs on an ongoing basis. Most significant incidents do not have one cause. Usually there are faults in the system, which are compounded by someone or several people being careless, tired, overworked or ill-informed. Cultivate an atmosphere of openness and discussion without blame so that you can all learn from the significant event. If people think they will be blamed they will hide the incident and no one will be able to prevent it happening again. Look for *all* the causes and try to remedy as many as possible to prevent the situation from arising in the future.

Evaluate the standards of care or services you provide

Keep your evaluation as simple as possible. Avoid wasting resources on unnecessarily bureaucratic evaluation. Design the evaluation so that you:

- specify the event (such as a service) to be evaluated – define broad issues, set priorities against strategic goals, time and resources, seek agreement on the nature and scope of the task

- describe the expected impact of the programme or activity and who will be affected
- define the criteria of success – these might relate to structure, process or outcome
- identify the information required to demonstrate the achievements of the programme or activity. The record might include: observing behaviour; data from existing records; prospective recording by the subjects of the programme or by the recipients and staff of the activity
- determine the time frame for the evaluation
- specify who collects the data for all stages in the delivery of the programme or activity, and the respective deadlines
- review and refine the objectives of the programme or activity and check that they are appropriate for the outcomes and impact you expect.

What to evaluate?

You could:

- adopt any, or all, of the six aspects of the health service's performance assessment framework (*see* Box 2.6)
- agree milestones and goals at stages in your programme or adopt others such as those relating to the National Service Frameworks for coronary heart disease or mental health
- evaluate the extent to which you achieve the outcome(s) starting with an objective. Alternatively, you might evaluate how conducive is the context of the programme, or activity, to achieving the anticipated outcomes
- undertake regular audits of aspects of the structure, process and outcome of a service or project to see if you have achieved what you expected when you established the criteria and standards of the audit programme
- evaluate the various components of a new system or programme: the activities, personnel involved, provision of services, organisational structure, precise goals and interventions.

Box 2.6: The six aspects of the NHS performance assessment framework

1 Health improvement
2 Fair access
3 Effective delivery
4 Efficiency
5 Patient/carer experience
6 Health outcomes

Computer search

The extent to which you can evaluate your practice will depend on the quality of your records and extent to which you use the capacity of your practice computer. Compare the results of a computerised search for all those using one type of treatment with another. Make appropriate changes to your systems depending on what the computer search reveals. Put your plan into action and monitor with repeat searches at regular intervals.

Look at your learning or service development needs by analysing data from practice records to:

- look at trends and patterns of illness
- devise and use clinical guidelines and decision support systems as part of evidence-based practice
- audit what you are doing
- provide the information on which to base decisions on commissioning and management
- support epidemiology, research and teaching activities.

Compare the systems in your practice with those required by legislation

Legislation changes quite frequently. As an employer, a GP needs to keep abreast of the legislation or ensure that the practice manager does so. You could start by comparing the systems in your practice with those required by the Disability Discrimination Act (1995) and health and safety legislation.

Consider your patient population's health needs

Create a detailed profile of your practice population. Ask your PCO or public health lead for information about your practice population and comparative information about the general population living in the district – morbidity and mortality statistics, referral patterns, age/sex mix, ethnicity, and population trends.

Include information about the wider determinants of health such as housing, numbers of the population in, and types of, employment, geographical location, the environment, crime and safety, educational attainment and socio-economic data. Make a note of any particular health problems such as higher than average teenage pregnancy rates or drug misuse. Focus on the current state of health inequalities within your practice population or between your practice population and the district as a whole. It may be that circumstances change, which in turn alters the proportion of minority groups in your practice population – such as if a continuing care home opens up in your practice area, or there is a flood of homeless people or asylum seekers into your locality.

Review teamwork

You can measure how effective the team is[23] – evaluate whether the team has:

- clear goals and objectives
- accountability and authority
- individual roles for members
- shared tasks
- regular internal formal and informal communication
- full participation by members
- confrontation of conflict
- feedback to individuals
- feedback about team performance
- outside recognition
- two-way external communication
- team rewards.

Assess the quality of your services

Quality may be subdivided into eight components: equity, access, acceptability and responsiveness, appropriateness, communication, continuity, effectiveness and efficiency.[12]

You might use the matrix in Box 2.7 as a way of ordering your approach to auditing a particular topic with the eight aspects of quality on the vertical axis and structure, process and outcome on the horizontal axis.[24] In this way you can generate up to 24 aspects of a particular topic. You might then focus on several aspects to look at the quality of patient care or services from various angles.

Look for service development needs reflecting why patients receive a poor quality of service such as:

- inadequately trained staff or staff with poor levels of competence
- lack of confidentiality
- staff not being trained in the management of emergency situations
- doctors or nurses not being contactable in an emergency or being ineffective
- treatment being unavailable due to poor management of resources or services
- poor management of the arrangements for home visiting

Box 2.7:   Matrix for assessing the quality of a clinical service

You might look at the structure, process or outcome of communicating test results to patients, for example:

	Structure	Process	Outcome
Equity			
Access			
Acceptability and responsiveness			
Appropriateness			
Communication	Hospital report	Feedback	Action taken
Continuity			
Effectiveness			
Efficiency			

- insufficient numbers of available staff for the workload
- qualifications of locums or deputising staff being unknown or inadequate for the posts they are filling
- arrangements for transfer of information from one team member to another being inadequate
- team members not acting on information received.

Many of these items will need action as a team, but for some of them, it may be your responsibility to ensure that adequate standards are met.

Reflect on whether you are providing cost-effective care and services

Cost-effectiveness is not synonymous with 'cheap'. A cost-effective intervention is one which gives a better or equivalent benefit from the intervention in question for lower or equivalent cost, or where the relative improvement in outcome is higher than the relative difference in cost. In other words being cost-effective means having the best outcomes for the least input. Using the term 'cost-effective' implies that you have considered potential alternatives.

An intervention must first be considered *clinically* effective to warrant investigation into its potential to be *cost*-effective. Evidence-based practice must incorporate clinical judgement. You have to interpret the evidence when it comes to applying it to individual patients, whether it is evidence about clinical effectiveness or cost-effectiveness. A new or alternative treatment or intervention should be compared directly with the previous best treatment or intervention.

An economic evaluation is a comparative analysis of two or more alternatives in terms of their costs and consequences. There are four different types as shown in Box 2.8.

Box 2.8:   The four types of economic evaluation

1   *Cost-effectiveness analysis* is used to compare the effectiveness of two interventions with the same treatment objectives
2   *Cost minimisation* compares the costs of alternative treatments that have identical health outcomes
3   *Cost–utility analysis* enables the effects of alternative interventions to be measured against a combination of life expectancy and quality of life; common outcome measures are quality adjusted life years (QALYs) or health-related quality of life (hrqol)
4   *Cost–benefit analysis* is a technique designed to determine the feasibility of a project, plan, management or treatment by quantifying its costs and benefits. It is often difficult to determine these accurately in relation to health.

While health valuation is unavoidable, it cannot be objective. You will probably have learning needs around what subjective method is best to use.[25]

Efficiency is sometimes confused with effectiveness. Being efficient means obtaining the most quality from the least expenditure, or the required level of quality for the least expenditure. To measure efficiency you need to make a judgement about the level of quality of the 'purchase' and be able to relate it to 'price'. 'Price' alone does not measure efficiency. Quality is the indicator used in combination with price to assess if something is more efficient. So, cost-effectiveness is a measure of efficiency and suggests that costs have been related to effectiveness.

Consider if you have service development needs. Discuss whether:

- the current skill mix in your team is appropriate
- more cost-effective alternative types of delivery of care are available
- sufficient staff training exists for those taking on new roles and responsibilities.

Set priorities: how you match what's needed with what's possible

You and your colleagues will have been able to make a wish list after following the previous Stages 3A and 3B undertaking a variety of needs assessments.

Group and summarise your learning and service development needs from the exercises you have carried out. Grade them according to the priority you set. You may put one at a higher priority because it fits in with learning needs established from another section, or put another lower because it does not fit in with other activities that you will put into your learning plan for the next 12 months. If you have identified a learning need by several different methods of assessment then it will have a higher priority than something only identified once in your PDP. Collect information from all the team, the patients, users and carers, to feed back before you make a decision on how to progress. Remember to take external influences into account such as the National Service Frameworks, National Institute for Clinical Excellence (NICE) guidance, governmental priorities, priorities of your PCO, the content of the Local Delivery Plan, etc.

Select those topics that are tied into organisational priorities, have clear aims and objectives and are achievable within your time and resource constraints. When ranking topics for learning or action in order of priority (Stage 4) consider whether:

- the project aims and objectives are clearly defined
- the topic is important:
  - for the population served (e.g. the size of the problem and/or its severity)
  - for the skills, knowledge or attitudes of the individual or team
- it is feasible
- it is affordable
- it will make enough difference
- it fits in with other priorities.

You will still have more ideas than can possibly be implemented. Remember the highest priority – the health service is for patients that use it or who will do so in the future.

References

1   Medical Professionalism Project (2002) Medical professionalism in the new millennium: a physicians' charter. *Lancet.* **359**: 520–2.

2   http://www.gpwsi.org/subindex.shtml.

3   Eraut M and du Boulay B (2000) *Developing the Attributes of Medical Professional Judgement and Competence.* University of Sussex, Sussex. Reproduced at http://www.cogs.susx.ac.uk/users/bend/doh.

4   Fraser SW and Greenhalgh T (2001) Coping with complexity: educating for capability. *British Medical Journal.* **323**: 799–802.

5   General Medical Council (2001) *Good Medical Practice.* General Medical Council, London.

6 Pendleton D, Schofield T, Tate P and Havelock P (2003) *The New Consultation, Developing Doctor–Patient Communication.* Oxford University Press, Oxford.

7 King J (2002) Career focus: 360° appraisal. *British Medical Journal.* **324**: S195.

8 Royal College of General Practitioners/General Practitioners' Committee (2002) *Good Medical Practice for General Practitioners.* Royal College of General Practitioners, London.

9 National Institute for Clinical Excellence (NICE) http://www.nice.org.uk.

10 Scottish Intercollegiate Guidelines Network (SIGN) http://www.sign.ac.uk.

11 Irvine D and Irvine S (eds) (1991) *Making Sense of Audit.* Radcliffe Medical Press, Oxford.

12 Maxwell RJ (1984) Quality assessment in health. *British Medical Journal.* **288**: 1470–2.

13 Toon P, Greenhalgh T, Rigby M *et al.* (2002) *The Human Face of Medicine.* Two CD ROMs in the APOLLO (Advancing Professional Practice through Online Learning Opportunities) series. BMJ Publishing Group, London. Free sample available at www.apollobmj.com.

14 *Guidelines in Practice* www.eguidelines.co.uk.

15 www.doctors.net.uk.

16 www.npcrdc.man.ac.uk.

17 http://latis.ex.ac.uk/cfep/index.htm.

18 Department of Health (2003) *EPP Update Newsletter.* Department of Health, London. See Expert Patient Programme on www.ohn.gov.uk/ohn/people/expert.htm.

19 Department of Health (2003) *The NHS Knowledge and Skills Framework (NHS KSF) and Development Review Guidance – working draft.* Version 6. Department of Health, London.

20 Department of Health (2003) *Job Evaluation Handbook.* Version 1. Department of Health, London.

21 Chambers R, Drinkwater C and Boath E (2003) *Involving Patients and the Public: how to do it better* (2e). Radcliffe Medical Press, Oxford.

22 Mohanna K and Chambers R (2000) *Risk Matters in Healthcare.* Radcliffe Medical Press, Oxford.

23 Hart E and Fletcher J (1999) Learning how to change: a selective analysis of literature and experience of how teams learn and organisations change. *Journal of Interprofessional Care.* **13(1)**: 53–63.

24 Firth-Cozens J (1993) *Audit in Mental Health Services.* LEA, Hove.

25 McCulloch D (2003) *Valuing Health in Practice.* Ashgate Publishing Ltd, Aldershot.

3

Demonstrating common components of good quality healthcare

In looking at the quality of care you provide and demonstrating your standards of service delivery and outcomes of learning, you should find that obtaining informed consent from patients for their treatment, maintaining confidentiality and handling complaints are part of the fabric of good quality care. We have considered them separately in this chapter, but each may be individualised to any of the seven clinical areas of Chapters 4 to 10.

We have set out the chapter with key information about consent followed by some example cycles of the stages of evidence (*see* Figure 1.1 on page 6). The two other sections on confidentiality and complaints follow, laid out in similar ways. Read through the cycles of evidence to become familiar with the approach to gathering and documenting evidence of your learning, competence, performance or standards of service delivery. Then either adopt one of the examples or adapt it to your own circumstances. Alternatively, read on to one or more of the clinical chapters and look at these three components in a clinical context such as in relation to contraception or sexually transmitted infections in Chapters 5 and 6.

Consent

Key points

Information given to a health professional remains the property of the patient. In most circumstances, consent is assumed for the necessary sharing of information with other professionals involved with the care of the patient for that episode of care. Usually consent is also assumed for essential sharing of information for continuing care. Beyond this, informed consent must be obtained. Patients attend for healthcare in the belief that the personal information that they supply, or which is found out about them during investigation or treatment, will be confidential.

Exceptions to the above are:[1]

- if the patient consents
- if it is in the patient's own interest that information should be disclosed, but it is either impossible to seek the patient's consent or
- it is medically undesirable in the patient's own interest, to seek the patient's consent
- if the law requires (and does not merely permit) the health professional to disclose the information
- if the health professional has an overriding duty to society to disclose the information
- if the health professional agrees with a governmental agency that disclosure is necessary to safeguard national security
- if the disclosure is necessary to prevent a serious risk to public health
- in certain circumstances, for the purposes of medical research.

Health professionals must be able to justify their decision to disclose information without consent. If they are in any doubt, they should consult their professional bodies and colleagues.

Consent is only valid if the patient fully understands the nature and consequences of disclosure – they must be able to give their consent, receive enough information to enable them to make a decision and be acting under their own free will and not persuaded by the strong influence of another person. If consent is given, the health worker is responsible for limiting the disclosure to that information for which informed consent has been obtained. The development of modern information technology and the increasing amount of multidisciplinary teamwork in patient care make confidentiality difficult to uphold.

You may need to give information about a patient to a relative or carer. Normally the consent of the patient should be obtained. Sometimes, the clinical condition of the patient may prevent informed consent being obtained (e.g. they are unconscious or have a severe illness). It is important to recognise that relatives or carers do *not* have any right to information about the patient. Disclosure without consent may be justified when third parties are exposed to a risk so serious that it outweighs the patient's privacy. An example would be if a patient declines to allow you to disclose information about their health and continues to drive against medical advice when unfit to do so.

Local research ethics committees and the research governance framework ensure best practice in the giving of informed consent by patients in research studies.

As health professionals, we often assume implied consent. The general public and patients are generally ignorant of the extent to which information about them is passed around the NHS. When teaching at both undergraduate and postgraduate levels, in examinations and assessments and in research, we may incorrectly assume patients imply their consent. Consent is also implied for health service accounting, central monitoring of referrals, in disease registers, for audit and in facilitating joint working between team members. The NHS is still engaged in a debate about what data can legitimately be shared without patients' explicit consent. Although written consent is usually obtained for supplying information to insurance companies or for legal reports, patients are often unaware of the type of information being supplied and have not given 'informed consent'. Guidelines published jointly by the British Medical Association (BMA) and the Association of British Insurers clarify that doctors are not required to release all aspects of a patient's medical history but need only submit (with the patient's consent) information that is relevant.[2]

The GMC's booklet *Seeking Patients' Consent: the ethical considerations* explores issues of consent in more depth and advises that:

the amount of information you give each patient will vary according to factors such as the nature of the condition, the complexity of the treatment, the risks associated with the treatment or procedure and the patient's own wishes ... you should be careful about relying on a patient's apparent compliance with a procedure as a form of consent.[3]

Collecting data to demonstrate your learning, competence, performance and standards of service delivery: consent

Example cycle of evidence 3.1

- Focus: informed consent
- Other relevant focus: relationships with patients

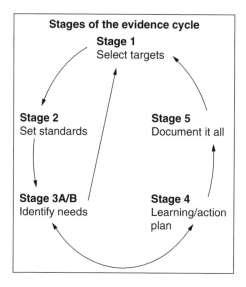

Stages of the evidence cycle

Stage 1
Select targets

Stage 2
Set standards

Stage 5
Document it all

Stage 3A/B
Identify needs

Stage 4
Learning/action plan

Box 3.1:   Case study

Mrs Bowed comes into surgery to see you about her contraception. You sketch out the alternatives that are open to her as a 35-year-old smoker. It transpires that she has had unprotected sexual intercourse four days previously and is at risk of pregnancy. You advise fitting an intrauterine device (IUD) straightaway, as this will provide emergency contraception and long-term contraception. 'You might as well – you know best,' she says passively, with a long sigh. Further discussion reveals that she felt pressured to have a termination of pregnancy by her mother when a teenager, with which the doctors colluded. Since then, she's never taken any real decisions about her health or contraception, having had a domineering husband who has recently left her.

This is just an example. Keep your task simple. You could choose three or four cycles of evidence to demonstrate your competence each year.

Stage 1: Select your aspirations for good practice

The excellent GP:

- obtains informed consent to treatment
- treats patients politely and with consideration.

Stage 2: Set the standards for your outcomes

Outcomes might include:

- the way learning is applied
- a learnt skill
- a protocol
- a strategy that is implemented
- meeting recommended standards.

- A completed audit that shows that you, or all clinicians in the team, consistently obtain women's informed consent to treatment or other clinical management.
- Devise, apply and act on an appropriate patient survey tool that ascertains patients' views about their treatment by yourself, other GPs or the practice team e.g. establishing views as to whether you treat patients politely and with consideration.
- You might choose to focus on referral for termination of pregnancy, or consent for contraception such as an injection, the fitting of an IUD or implant, or for investigations such as taking vaginal swabs.

Stage 3A: Identify your learning needs

- Review the consent and communication issues in a complaint or expression of discontent made by a patient to any member of the practice team.
- Reflect on whether you follow best practice in obtaining and recording consent to treatment or procedures.

Stage 3B: Identify your service needs

> Any of the needs assessment exercises in 3A may also reveal service needs.

- Compare the consent policy in your practice against recommended best practice or another practice's consent policy and reflect on the differences.
- Audit the case notes to determine whether doctors and nurses recorded the discussion of parental knowledge and consent to treatment with contraception in consultations with under-16 year olds.
- Undertake a targeted teenage patient survey. You might look at teenagers who have consulted GPs or nurses at the surgery. Alternatively, you might learn more from a survey of teenagers at a local youth centre, as this would include non-users of GP services. You could ask about any aspect of teenage health, such as their experiences of informed consent, or how treatment options have been explained, or their experience of consultations with local GPs or nurses, relating to politeness and consideration.

Stage 4: Make and carry out a learning and action plan

- Identify the issues from the learning and service needs assessment exercises in Stages 3A and 3B, e.g. comparing your own consent policy with others.
- Set up a workshop on communication skills highlighting politeness and consideration, and ability to gain informed consent, e.g. by video recording and reflection/feedback with various types of patients including teenagers.
- Arrange and attend a facilitated meeting with a group of women to discuss their experiences of consulting GPs and the practice, to gain their opinions about access, the welcome, and general attitudes in the surgery e.g. organised by the practice's patient participation group.

Stage 5: Document your learning, competence, performance and standards of service delivery

- Make notes of the review of the complaint or adverse comments and subsequent plan to minimise likelihood of re-occurrence.
- Repeat the initial learning or service needs assessments, e.g. re-audit and repeat the patient survey.
- Audit that the consent policy is applied consistently by all clinical members of the practice team, e.g. from case notes, patient feedback, self-report. You might find that consent is reported as being obtained but not recorded in the patients' records. This would imply that a change in recording practice is required and produce future new learning needs!

Box 3.2:   Case study continued

You help Mrs Bowed to understand the risk and consequences of pregnancy and the urgency of action she needs to take if she wishes to receive emergency contraception. You talk through the advantages and disadvantages of the fitting of an IUD and its use as long-term contraception. You suggest an assert-iveness course run by the local further education college she might like to consider. You fit the IUD after surgery later the same day when she has had an opportunity to reflect about what she wants to do and has given informed consent to the fitting.

Example cycle of evidence 3.2

- Focus: informed consent
- Other relevant focus: research

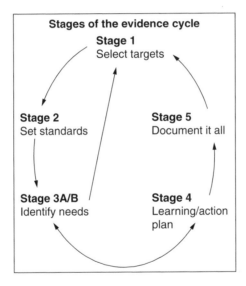

Box 3.3:   Case study

You agree as a practice to undertake a survey to find out if patients are satisfied with your service. The practice manager will organise it, but you are nominated to lead the work. You decide to focus on teenagers as a group as the adolescent drop-in clinic you set up two years ago with the school health service is not being used as much as it once was. You are not sure how to survey the teenagers. You think they are unlikely to answer questionnaires sent through the post and think you will interview teenagers about their satisfaction with the clinic. You intend to employ one of your own teenage children to interview some who have never come to the clinic, by selecting their names from your patient list, as well as some teenagers who have attended. You're not sure if you are getting into research territory or if it is okay to claim you are auditing your services.

> This is just an example. Keep your task simple. You could choose three or four cycles of evidence to demonstrate your competence each year.

Stage 1: Select your aspirations for good practice

The excellent GP:

- protects patients' rights and makes sure that they are not disadvantaged by taking part in research
- gives patients the information they need about their problem in a way they can understand as a basis for informed consent.

Stage 2: Set the standards for your outcomes

Outcomes might include:

- the way learning is applied
- a learnt skill
- a protocol
- a strategy that is implemented
- meeting recommended standards.

- Informed consent policy of practice covers patients' participation in audit and research as well as consent to clinical treatment.
- You should be able to describe the difference between audit of clinical management and service provision and research.

Stage 3A: Identify your learning needs

- Read through the frequently asked questions and answers on the Department of Health website relating to research governance.[4] Consider whether you are able to answer the questions before reading the answers.
- Describe an audit plan of an adolescent clinic that involves obtaining young people's views of standards of services by interviewing them. Submit the plan to the chair of the local research ethics committee to check that he/she agrees that the audit proposal does not fall within the definition of research and to approve the patient literature and the process inviting informed consent to take part.

Stage 3B: Identify your service needs

Any of the needs assessment exercises in 3A may also reveal service needs.

- Draw up an information leaflet for young people about the audit of adolescent clinic services that you intend to carry out. Ask others to critique the leaflet – young people for its readability and clarity, a research colleague for the extent to which it conforms to best practice for informed consent. Use the information leaflet so that they can give informed consent to the interview to obtain their views and audio recording of the interview.
- Ask a colleague to peer review the extent to which advice and information you give to teenagers during a consultation is accurate. The teenager would need to have given prior, written informed consent for the peer review (and audio recording if used).

Stage 4: Make and carry out a learning and action plan

- Obtain and read documents about research governance from the Department of Health's website[4] or from your PCO – as in section 3A (first point).
- Study the application form for the ethical approval of a research study.
- Understand the limits to obtaining patients' views as part of audit of clinical and service management by reading up on informed consent. Read the GMC's booklet: *Seeking Patients' Consent: the ethical considerations.*[3] Look

at whether you are explaining the details of the diagnosis or prognosis, giving an explanation of likely benefits and side-effects, explaining whether a proposed treatment is experimental and whether a doctor in training will be involved.
- Ask for a short tutorial from your local clinical governance lead about good practice in obtaining patients' views through audit, research and patient involvement activities – including good practice in informed consent.

Stage 5: Document your learning, competence, performance and standards of service delivery

- Make a comparison of your own practice with the answers to the frequently asked questions on the Department of Health website relating to research governance.[4]
- File a response letter from the chair of the local research ethics committee about the audit proposal.
- Keep the subsequent revised audit plan to ensure that work does not fall within the definition of research.
- Keep the revised patients' informed consent leaflet, following the critique.
- Repeat the peer review by the same, or another, colleague of the extent to which advice and information you give to teenagers during consultations is accurate.

Box 3.4:   Case study continued

The chair of the research ethics committee advises you that your plan should be classed as research rather than audit as it involves contact with patients outside their usual NHS care. He explains about the risks of using untrained interviewers such as your own children and the need to fully inform those teenagers you are inviting to be interviewed about the survey, and that their refusal will not prejudice their medical care. He advises you to send an application form for formal approval to the ethics committee and to contact the research lead in your PCO in line with the research governance framework if you wish to continue to develop a research project. You revise your plans as the scale of the work required is becoming out of all proportion.

Example cycle of evidence 3.3

- Focus: informed consent
- Other relevant focus: working with colleagues

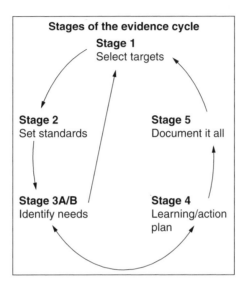

Stages of the evidence cycle

Stage 1
Select targets

Stage 2
Set standards

Stage 5
Document it all

Stage 3A/B
Identify needs

Stage 4
Learning/action plan

Box 3.5: Case study

Miss Young comes with her carer to see you. The carer explains that the new manager of the unit for people with learning disabilities, in which Miss Young lives, wants Miss Young to have a cervical smear and mammography. Although Miss Young is 52 years old she has had neither screening test. You wonder how to proceed, as Miss Young does not seem to have any say in this.

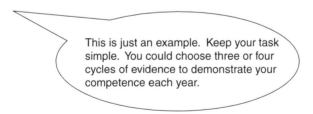

This is just an example. Keep your task simple. You could choose three or four cycles of evidence to demonstrate your competence each year.

Stage 1: Select your aspirations for good practice

The excellent GP:

- acts in the best interests of patients when making referrals and providing or arranging treatment or care, acting with patients' informed consent

- makes sure that others understand their professional status and speciality, what roles and responsibilities they have and who is responsible for each aspect of the patient's care.

Stage 2: Set the standards for your outcomes

Outcomes might include:
- the way learning is applied
- a learnt skill
- a protocol
- a strategy that is implemented
- meeting recommended standards.

- Publish a practice policy on informed consent for patients with mental health problems and learning disabilities, including dementia.

Stage 3A: Identify your learning needs

- Analyse a significant event, e.g. you referred Miss Young for mammography and she refuses to co-operate in the X-ray department resulting in a telephoned protest from the radiographer.
- Self-assessment – you are aware that you do not know how to proceed (e.g. in the consultation in the case study). You do not know how much you can rely on the carer having already gained Miss Young's informed consent or the extent to which you can take Miss Young's acquiescence for 'consent'.
- Read up and reflect on the association between competency or capacity to be well informed and the degree of previous education and the inability of some individuals to provide informed consent, if they have educational, social and cultural reasons that limit their understanding of complex issues.

Stage 3B: Identify your service needs

Any of the needs assessment exercises in 3A may also reveal service needs.

- Carry out a review of case notes of women aged 20–65 years old with learning disabilities to determine the numbers who have had cervical smears, mammograms, immunisations, etc.

- Arrange a focus group discussion with people with learning disabilities and their carers (or other target group such as people with dementia and their carers) to discuss the appropriateness of the patient's consent process for all clinical interventions including cervical cytology and mammography.

Stage 4: Make and carry out a learning and action plan

- Ask advice from MENCAP about the approach they recommend for obtaining informed consent from 'vulnerable' groups of people, how to explain clinical management and pursue clinical interventions, together with any associated useful literature.
- Read up on informed consent.
- Revise the practice informed consent policy to include specific groups of 'vulnerable' people such as those with learning disabilities or mental ill-health problems.

Stage 5: Document your learning, competence, performance and standards of service delivery

- Run a quiz for members of the practice team at an in-house educational event with four hypothetical cases. Compare the answers with best practice according to MENCAP[5] and other professional literature.
- Include the revised practice policy on informed consent.
- Audit the consistent application of the revised practice informed consent policy with consecutive cases, e.g. search on people coded as having learning disability on computer. Look to see what interventions have been undertaken and whether informed consent has been recorded in the notes.
- Use specimen consent forms that have been piloted, revised and audited.

Box 3.6: Case study continued

Miss Young returns for a follow-up appointment, having been left at the last surgery appointment to think about having a cervical smear and with a referral for mammography. She has told her carer that she has had some bleeding from down below so a pelvic examination and smear are warranted clinically. You take plenty of time to explain how you will do the pelvic examination and smear, Miss Young agrees and all goes well.

Confidentiality

Key points

You should have appropriate confidentiality safeguards in place in the practice to prevent inadvertent disclosure of personal and sensitive information about patients. Tell people, especially the young, about their right to confidential medical treatment and reinforce your conversation with posters and leaflets. People with non-prescription drug-related problems who seek help from substance abuse clinics, or those with sexually transmitted infections who attend genitourinary medicine clinics, often do not want their GP to be told because they do not believe that the information will be kept confidential. Fears about confidentiality are the commonest reason young people give for not attending their GP for contraceptive treatment.[6]

Young people under the age of 16 years have the same rights to confidentiality as other patients. The younger the person, the greater the care that is needed to assess the level of understanding to ensure that he or she understands the consequences of any proposed action. If a young person fulfils the conditions given in Box 3.7 he or she is regarded as being competent to make his or her own decisions.

Box 3.7: The Fraser Guidelines[7]

The guidelines were drawn up after Lord Fraser stated in 1985 that a doctor could give contraceptive advice or treatment to a person under 16 years old without parental consent, providing that the doctor is satisfied that:

- the young person will understand the advice
- the young person cannot be persuaded to tell their parents or allow the doctor to tell them that they are seeking contraceptive advice
- the young person is likely to begin or continue having unprotected sex with or without contraceptive treatment
- the young person's physical or mental health is likely to suffer unless they receive contraceptive advice or treatment
- it is in the young person's best interest to receive contraceptive advice or treatment.

The Fraser Guidelines apply to health professionals in England and Wales. In Scotland, the Age of Legal Capacity (Scotland) Act 1991 gives similar powers of consent to those under 16 years of age.

In Northern Ireland, although separate legislation applies, the then Department of Health and Social Services Northern Ireland stated that there was no reason to suppose that the House of Lords' decision would not be followed by the Northern Ireland Courts.

Occasionally you may feel that you have a moral obligation to divulge confidential information. Whenever possible you should seek to persuade the patient to give consent to the disclosure. Seek advice from your professional organisations in circumstances where others are in danger (e.g. risk of harm, or rape or sexual abuse), or where a serious crime has been committed. Health professionals should satisfy themselves that sufficient authority has been obtained (e.g. a certificate from the Attorney General or Lord Advocate) and consult professional organisations before disclosing information without a patient's consent.

Box 3.8:   The Caldicott Committee Report

The Caldicott Committee Report described principles of good practice to safeguard confidentiality when information is being used for non-clinical purposes:[8]

- justify the purpose
- do not use patient-identifiable information unless it is absolutely necessary
- use the minimum necessary patient-identifiable information
- access to patient-identifiable information should be on a strict need-to-know basis
- everyone with access to patient-identifiable information should be aware of his or her responsibilities.

Interpreters should be used wherever possible to avoid the use of friends or relatives. They should be trained in the requirements of confidentiality.

Patients are entitled to access data held about them. Exceptions to this right are:

- the patient failed to make the request in accordance with the Data Protection Act 1998
- if acceding to the request would result in disclosure of information about somebody else without their consent
- when giving medical information may cause serious harm to the mental or physical health of the patient (a rare occurrence).

You need to incorporate systems for ensuring that paper and computer security are maintained. Systems for monitoring and upgrading security systems should be in place and you should check regularly that confidentiality is not being breached if changes are made.

Collecting data to demonstrate your learning, competence, performance and standards of service delivery: confidentiality

Example cycle of evidence 3.4

- Focus: confidentiality
- Other relevant focus: teaching and training

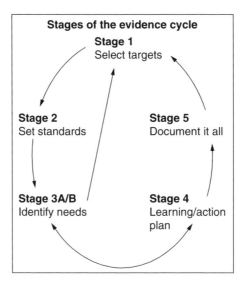

Stages of the evidence cycle

Stage 1
Select targets

Stage 2
Set standards

Stage 5
Document it all

Stage 3A/B
Identify needs

Stage 4
Learning/action plan

Box 3.9:   Case study

It is the first time you have had students placed with you and you want to teach two of them about the importance of making sure that young people understand the practice code on confidentiality while they are on their placement with you.

This is just an example. Keep your task simple. You could choose three or four cycles of evidence to demonstrate your competence each year.

Stage 1: Select your aspirations for good practice

The excellent GP:

- maintains the confidentiality of patient-specific information
- ensures that patients are not put at risk when seeing students or doctors in training.

Stage 2: Set the standards for your outcomes

> Outcomes might include:
>
> - the way learning is applied
> - a learnt skill
> - a protocol
> - a strategy that is implemented
> - meeting recommended standards.

- Ensure that all members of the practice team including you, new members of staff and students or doctors in training are familiar with guidelines for confidentiality in relation to patients receiving healthcare.

Stage 3A: Identify your learning needs

- Assess your knowledge about the limits of confidentiality, e.g. for providing under-16 year olds with contraception or referring them for termination of pregnancy or other surgical intervention.
- Ask an expert tutor's opinion about the particular method of teaching you plan to use for an in-house training session on maintaining confidentiality for teenagers of different ages that will best convey main messages and lead to changes where necessary.

Stage 3B: Identify your service needs

> Any of the needs assessment exercises in 3A may also reveal service needs.

- Compare the practice protocol for confidentiality with the guidelines in the *Confidentiality and Young People* toolkit.[6]
- Review the intended induction programme for new members of staff, students on placement and doctors in training to assess the extent to which knowledge of confidentiality features and is addressed.

Stage 4: Make and carry out a learning and action plan

- Find out from the local educational tutor how to undertake learning needs assessments of others from different disciplines with different levels of responsibilities in respect of confidentiality.
- Prepare for and run an interactive teaching session on confidentiality for patients of all age groups with special focus on teenagers. You might invite the whole practice team, including students, family planning or school nurses, local pharmacists, GP registrars, etc. You could use the *Confidentiality and Young People* toolkit for promoting discussion with the practice team at the session.[6]

Stage 5: Document your learning, competence, performance and standards of service delivery

- Run a quiz completed by those attending the teaching session before and after training about confidentiality.
- Create an incident record kept by the practice team of any reported or perceived breaches of confidentiality by anyone working in, or associated with, the practice.
- Ensure the existence of personal learning plans based on learning needs assessments for new staff or doctors in training by the end of their induction period.
- Revise the practice protocol in line with the *Confidentiality and Young People* toolkit.

Box 3.10:   Case study continued

Other staff colleagues join your teaching session with the students using the video from the *Confidentiality and Young People* toolkit.[6] All get full marks in the quiz after watching the video.

Learning from complaints

Key points

There is learning to be had from every complaint. The GMC received a record 5539 complaints in 2002, 4% more than in 2001; of these, 72 resulted in a doctor being banned or suspended.[9] Even if the complaint is trivial or undeserved, it implies a lack of communication. Table 3.1 describes the nature of claims against GPs reported in a study of 1000 consecutive clinical cases. There are a myriad of associated reasons for the claims. Many of the clinical events will reveal failings in the practice systems and processes and in the practice of the GP – such as communication, diagnostic skills, etc.

Table 3.1:   The nature of 1000 claims against GPs handled by the Medical Protection Society[10]

Claim by patient	Number of claims
Problems of diagnosis (delayed or missed)	631
Prescribing errors	193
Malignant neoplasms (some of the problems of diagnosis)	140
Cancer of the breast (lumpiness often falsely diagnosed as benign)	20
Cancer of the cervix (often abnormalities filed away and not acted upon)	14
Cancer of the digestive organs (cancer of the colon most frequent with misdiagnosed symptoms)	21
Diabetes (8 deaths) primary failure to diagnose (19 delays in diagnosis) (9 delays in referral of patient resulting in amputation)	40
Myocardial infarction 27 deaths (8 undiagnosed, 7 diagnosed as dyspepsia, 3 diagnosed as congestive cardiac failure, 3 as muscular origin, 2 as chest infection)	34
Prescribing	
Steroids (e.g. osteoporotic collapse)	40
Antibiotic allergy	8
Phenothiazines (extrapyramidal symptoms)	10
Hormone replacement therapy	9
Oral contraception	9
Warfarin (interactions e.g. resulting in cerebral haemorrhage)	5

Collecting data to demonstrate your learning, competence, performance and standards of service delivery: complaints

Example cycle of evidence 3.5

- Focus: complaints
- Other relevant focus of evidence: working with colleagues

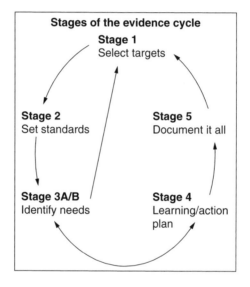

Stages of the evidence cycle

Stage 1
Select targets

Stage 2
Set standards

Stage 5
Document it all

Stage 3A/B
Identify needs

Stage 4
Learning/action plan

Box 3.11:   Case study

Your practice has received a patient complaint about a GP locum failing to diagnose a patient's bowel cancer on the first occasion they consulted. This has prompted you all as a practice team to review the way that your complaints system functions.

This is just an example. Keep your task simple. You could choose three or four cycles of evidence to demonstrate your competence each year.

Stage 1: Select your aspirations for good practice

The excellent GP:

- apologises appropriately when things go wrong, and has an adequate complaints procedure in place.

Stage 2: Set the standards for your outcomes

Outcomes might include:

- the way learning is applied
- a learnt skill
- a protocol
- a strategy that is implemented
- meeting recommended standards.

- Understand and establish effective processes for preventing and managing complaints from patients in the practice.

Stage 3A: Identify your learning needs

- Examine as a significant event one or more complaints, e.g. where the practice has not advised a patient correctly about the complaints process.
- Compare the actual care of a patient against an acceptable standard of care for a range of clinical conditions as ongoing review for a clinical area that has been the subject of a complaint (e.g. bowel cancer in case study). You could use peer review by asking respected colleagues or compare your practice against a published standard such as a guideline by a responsible body of professional opinion.

Stage 3B: Identify your service needs

Any of the needs assessment exercises in 3A may also reveal service needs.

- Audit patient complaints in the preceding 12 months: the number, the outcomes and how the complaint system is advertised, etc.
- Audit the extent to which doctors and nurses are following practice-agreed protocols. This is about being proactive about preventing or minimising the likelihood of the source of the complaint recurring.

- Audit vulnerable areas. Look back at the analysis of complaints to identify useful areas for focusing learning, e.g. a review of the prescribing of steroids.
- Review the way that the qualifications of locums are checked and that they are made aware of the practice protocols.

Stage 4: Make and carry out a learning and action plan

- Ask your PCO to look at the practice complaints system and feed back how it can be improved (if at all).
- Arrange a tutorial between the practice manager and others in the team about preventing and managing complaints, or use one of the risk management packages produced by medical defence organisations.[11,12]
- Read up on how to undertake significant event analysis including how to share the information with the practice team and respond as a practice team.

Stage 5: Document your learning, competence, performance and standards of service delivery

- Collect evidence of clinical competence to guard against a complaint.
- Develop a protocol of the patient complaint process against which consecutive complaints can be audited in another 12 months' time.
- Document guidance about physical examinations including that the reason for any examination should be communicated clearly, that a chaperone should be offered for any internal or breast examination, and the comfort and privacy of the patient should always be kept in mind to avoid potential complaints.
- Make sure a file containing practice protocols is available for easy reference on the desktop of the computer.

Box 3.12:   Case study continued

You are invited by your PCO to take a lead in advising GPs in other practices about the handling of complaints because they were impressed by the way your complaint system was applied when you invited them to visit your practice and advise about the handling of complaints.

References

1   Chambers R and Wakley G (2000) *Making Clinical Governance Work for You.* Radcliffe Medical Press, Oxford.

2   British Medical Association and Association of British Insurers (2002) *Medical Information and Insurance.* British Medical Association, London (*see* www.bma.org.uk/ap.nsf/Content/MedicalInfoInsurance).

3   General Medical Council (2002) *Seeking Patients' Consent: the ethical considerations.* General Medical Council, London.

4   www.doh.gov.uk/research/.

5   http://www.mencap.org.uk.

6   Royal College of General Practitioners and Brook (2000) *Confidentiality and Young People. A toolkit for general practice, primary care groups and trusts.* Royal College of General Practitioners, London.

7   The Fraser Guidelines (1985) House of Lords Judgement, London.

8   Department of Health (1997) Report of the Review of Patient-identifiable Information. In: *The Caldicott Committee Report.* Department of Health, London.

9   General Medical Council (2003) *Fitness to Practise Statistics for 2002.* General Medical Council, London.

10 Panting G (2003) *Nature of 1000 Claims against GPs.* Medical Protection Society, London (presentation at primary care conference, Birmingham).

11 MPS Risk Consulting, Granary Wharf House, Leeds LS11 5PY or http://www.mps-riskconsulting.com.

12 MDU Services Ltd, 230 Blackfriars Road, London SE1 8PJ or http://www.the-mdu.com.

4

Women's health and lifestyle

Box 4.1: Case study

Mrs Hart comes to see you to ask for a 'well woman' check. Before you advise her to book in with the practice nurse for such a check, you ask her what has precipitated her request. She becomes tearful and tells you that one of her closest friends has just had a heart attack and died and that has made Mrs Hart worry about the damage her own unhealthy lifestyle might be doing. You look at her – an obese woman who looks older than her 48 years, no doubt from her longstanding smoking habit. She confesses that she drinks a half or full bottle of red wine most days and rarely takes any exercise but declares that she is careful not to eat excess fat. You refer her to the practice nurse for the 'well woman' check and counselling about her lifestyle habits and arrange to see her for follow up with the results of her fasting lipid profile and other screening tests.

What issues you should cover

Cigarette smoking[1]

Approximately 10 million adults in the UK are cigarette smokers and a similar number are ex-smokers. There is no significant difference between the numbers of men and women who smoke. Cigarette smoking is more common among those employed in manual jobs compared with those employed in professional and other non-manual occupations.

About 20% of all deaths in the UK population are attributable to smoking. About half of all regular cigarette smokers will die prematurely because of their smoking habit, and a quarter of regular smokers die before the age of 70 years. It costs the NHS around £1500 million to treat patients with smoking-related diseases each year. Mrs Hart needs to understand the risks that she is running from her longstanding smoking habit – especially from lung cancer, bronchitis and emphysema and coronary heart disease – and what she has to gain from stopping smoking. About a third of deaths from cancers of all kinds can be attributed to cigarette smoking. Cigarette smoking is the most important modifiable, non-genetic risk factor for coronary heart disease, and accounts for 11% of all heart disease deaths in women. Smoking during pregnancy is associated with an increased risk of spontaneous abortion, haemorrhage, premature birth and low birth weight as well as many problems with the infant following birth. Smoking is also associated with infertility and subfertility in women and men.

If Mrs Hart can be persuaded to stop smoking, the risks of ill-health induced by her cigarette smoking will soon fall. After one year, her risk of a heart attack will fall to about half that of a smoker; after ten years of not smoking, her risk of lung cancer is reduced to about half that of a smoker. After 15 years of not smoking, her risk of a heart attack will be the same as if she had never smoked.

The practice nurse should warn Mrs Hart about the withdrawal symptoms she may experience when she ceases to smoke. In most people, these include irritability or aggression, depression, restlessness, impaired concentration, increased appetite and craving for cigarettes. Mrs Hart may also experience light-headedness and disturbed sleep.

Psychological and behavioural techniques are key to helping patients to stop smoking. The practice nurse may have these skills and be trained in smoking cessation support. If so, Mrs Hart should learn to feel that she is capable of successfully stopping smoking (self-efficacy) and recognise and quash cues in her environment that will trigger cravings to smoke again. The fact that Mrs Hart is worried about her own risks from smoking following her friend's death means that health messages about stopping smoking should have a maximal impact upon her at this time. Combining psychological and behavioural counselling or group support with pharmacological interventions such as nicotine replacement or bupropion therapy increases smoking cessation rates so that as many as nearly one in five ex-smokers are still abstaining from smoking, six months after giving up. However, longer-term follow up studies show that many ex-smokers go on to relapse and start smoking again.

Acupuncture and hypnotherapy are both thought to be helpful although there is little research evidence about their effectiveness.

The six 'A's is a recommended approach for those in primary care to help patients like Mrs Hart to stop smoking.[1] That is, *ask* about smoking at every consultation, *advise* about risks and benefits of stopping smoking, *assess* the patient's willingness to quit smoking, *assist* the patient in planning to stop smoking, *arrange* follow up and *audit* the practice team's success in helping patients to stop.

Many health professionals are familiar with the well known staged approach[2] where patients are assessed for their readiness to change, and smoking cessation interventions are tailored to the stage patients have reached.[3] Conclusions from a systematic review[3] were that, overall, stage-based interventions are no more effective than non-stage-based interventions or no intervention, in changing smoking behaviour.

You and the practice nurse should be aware that smoking is a coping mechanism for many smokers like Mrs Hart who may believe that cigarettes calm them down if they are worried or anxious. Many smokers will have tried unsuccessfully to give up in the past – and you will be trying to motivate Mrs Hart to quit smoking despite her feeling powerless to give up because of her past failures to do so.

Obesity

You or the practice nurse will establish whether Mrs Hart is overweight or obese before advising her about risks to her health and treatment options. Overweight and obesity are most commonly defined by clinicians in terms of the body mass index (BMI).[4] The BMI is calculated as: weight in kilogrammes/ (height in metres)^2.

Overweight is generally classed as having a BMI between 25 and 29.9 and obesity as having a BMI of 30 or over. BMI does not distinguish between mass due to body fat and muscles. Nor does it take account of the distribution of fat around the body. Some individuals who might not be defined as obese according to their BMIs may still have a high degree of abdominal obesity, also termed 'central' obesity. Central obesity is measured by the waist circumference or by the waist to hip ratio. The relative distribution of fat between waist and hip predicts subsequent coronary artery disease better than body mass index. There are increased health risks from obesity when the waist circumference exceeds 94 cm for men and 80 cm for women.[5] You will probably find that Mrs Hart has a BMI over 30 and a waist circumference of more than 80 cm if she looks obese to you.

Mrs Hart is one of many who are overweight or obese. The UK has the fastest growing rate of obesity in Europe, almost trebling in the past 20 years. Thirty-three per cent of adult women are overweight and another 20% are obese. Men have similar problems, with 45% being overweight and another 17% being obese.[6]

Ask Mrs Hart if she indulges in 'binge eating' – a pattern that may be present in 20–30% of people who are obese. Binge eating is eating an amount of food that is larger than most people would eat in a similar time period under similar circumstances. Ask about her typical food intake – does she accept she is eating too much, or is physically inactive? It is common for obese and over-weight people to underestimate their food intake by about a third – perhaps because of genuine forgetfulness or self-deception or a lack of understanding of food composition, particularly hidden fat. In particular, people under-report their eating of snacks when they are totting up what they have eaten in a day.

Warn Mrs Hart about the risks to her health from her obesity. Obesity leads to premature mortality – there are lots of facts given in Tables 4.1 and 4.2 that you can relay to Mrs Hart. For instance, the risk of a fatal or non-fatal myocardial infarction among women with a BMI greater than 29 is three times that of lean women after adjustment for age and smoking.[7] Table 4.1 lists the proportion of various health problems that can be attributed to overweight or obesity. Mrs Hart might be impressed by the figures for the relative risks she is running of diabetes, hypertension, myocardial infarction and other clinical conditions compared to a woman who is not obese – try quoting some of the statistics to her listed in Table 4.2.

Tell Mrs Hart about the likely benefits to her health from losing weight. Specific examples can be impressive. For instance, in one study of 1200 people whose BMIs were between 25 and 37 and none of whom were being treated for hypertension, those who had lost at least 4.5 kg of weight by six months had an initial average fall in systolic and diastolic blood pressures of 8 or 9 mmHg that was maintained at follow up 36 months later. The lower levels of blood pressure at six months were not maintained at follow up in those who failed to sustain the 4.5 kg or more weight loss at six months.[8] There is now consistent evidence that weight loss not only reduces blood pressure in people who are overweight and hypertensive, but also in those who are overweight with high-normal blood pressure.

Table 4.1: Proportion of various conditions attributable to excess weight (BMI >27 kg/m²)[7]

Disease	Number out of 100 people
Hypertension	24.1
Myocardial infarction	13.9
Angina pectoris	20.5
Stroke	25.8
Venous thrombosis	7.7
Type 2 diabetes	24.1
Hyperlipidaemia	7.7
Gout	20.0
Osteoarthritis	11.8
Gall bladder disease	14.3
Colorectal cancer	4.7
Breast cancer	3.2
Genitourinary cancer	9.1

Table 4.2: Relative risks of different health problems in obese versus non-obese people[6]

Condition	Relative risk	
	Women	Men
Type 2 diabetes	12.7	5.2
Hypertension	4.2	2.6
Heart attack	3.2	1.5
Colon cancer	2.7	3.0
Angina	1.8	1.8
Gall bladder disease	1.8	1.8
Ovarian cancer	1.7	
Osteoarthritis	1.4	1.9
Stroke	1.3	1.3

The risk for a non-obese person is taken as 1 and the relative risks of an obese person developing the conditions are given in comparison for men and women

A 10% loss of body weight over the course of one year is a realistic target for most people. Box 4.2 describes the range of benefits to Mrs Hart's health she could expect if she lost 10% of her body weight in the next 12 months.

Mrs Hart may ask for advice about diet. There has been a great deal of recent interest in the efficacy of low carbohydrate diets. A systematic review concluded that there was insufficient evidence to make recommendations for

---

Box 4.2: Benefits of 10% loss of body weight in an obese person[9]

Mortality
More than 20% decrease in premature mortality
More than 30% decrease in diabetes-related deaths

Blood pressure
10 mmHg decrease in systolic blood pressure
20 mmHg decrease in diastolic blood pressure

Diabetes
50% decrease in fasting glucose

Lipids
30% decrease in triglycerides
10% decrease in total cholesterol
15% decrease in low density lipoprotein (LDL) cholesterol
8% increase in high density lipoprotein (HDL) cholesterol

or against the use of low carbohydrate diets. Weight loss among obese people was associated with longer diet duration and decreased calorie intake rather than the carbohydrate content of their diet. Low carbohydrate diets appeared to have no significant adverse effects on serum lipids, fasting glucose or insulin levels or blood pressure in one study.[10] Another reviewer concluded that the choice of diet

> may come down to suitably matching a dietary regimen to an individual's taste. For some of us a high protein diet with bacon and eggs, steak, fish and cheese would be heaven. For others, purgatory. Perhaps now people who want or need to lose weight have more of a choice about what might best suit them.[11]

Mrs Hart may feel that she cannot lose weight without additional help and so ask about drug therapy. Drug treatment should always be combined with diet and behaviour management.

Patients should show that they are motivated by losing at least 2.5 kg over a four week period before being prescribed drug treatment.

Drug therapy available to obese patients includes:

- orlistat (Xenical) which decreases fat absorption by inhibiting the enzyme lipase
- sibutramine (Reductil), a serotonin and noradrenaline reuptake inhibitor.

You will need to be able to explain to Mrs Hart the advantages and disadvantages of drug therapy and the commitment she will be making to maintaining weight loss through dietary control and increased physical activity. Medication is used as an adjunct to dietary, lifestyle and behavioural therapies in patients with sufficient motivation to adhere to an appropriate dietary regime.

Criteria for prescribing orlistat in line with NICE guidelines are given in Box 4.3. Orlistat is used in conjunction with a mildly hypocaloric diet containing around a third of calories from fat. Orlistat has an optimum effect at a dose of 120 mg three times a day. It is taken before, during or up to an hour after each main meal and the dose is omitted if a meal is missed or contains no fat.[12] Adverse effects such as oily spotting from the rectum, flatulence and faecal urgency occur in up to 27% of people taking orlistat.[13]

Box 4.3:   Criteria for prescribing orlistat[14]

- The licensing criteria and the NICE recommendations require potential patients to lose 2.5 kg in the month preceding the first prescription for orlistat, by dietary control and increased physical activity. This indicates whether a person is able to maintain a suitably low fat intake and reasonable amount of physical activity.

continued opposite

- Patients should have documented evidence of a BMI of 30 and above or a BMI of 28 and above with significant co-morbidity such as type 2 diabetes, hypertension or dyslipidaemia.
- Patients taking orlistat should be offered specific concomitant advice, support and counselling on diet, physical activity and behavioural strategies.
- People taking orlistat should be monitored and weighed on a monthly basis and thereafter as part of a supervised weight management plan.
- People continuing to be prescribed orlistat should have 5% weight loss at three months from the start of drug treatment and at least 10% cumulative weight loss at six months from the start of treatment.
- Treatment should not be continued beyond 12 months, and never beyond 24 months.
- The medication can only be prescribed for adults aged 18 to 75 years.

NICE guidance is similar in recommending that sibutramine should only be prescribed for people who have seriously attempted to lose weight by diet, exercise and other behavioural modifications, and that those prescribed the drug should be offered specific support, advice and counselling on these factors.[12,15] Sibutramine should only be used for people in the same category of risk from their overweight or obesity as for orlistat (*see* Box 4.3). Sibutramine creates a feeling of satiety by acting as a serotonin and noradrenaline reuptake inhibitor in the brain, enabling patients to feel satisfied after eating smaller quantities of food. It may also increase thermogenesis by stimulant action on the peripheral noradrenergic system. Monitoring of treatment is essential (*see* Box 4.4). Weight loss is maximal over the first six months and continues at a slower rate thereafter.[16] Sibutramine can reduce total cholesterol and triglycerides, with an increase in HDL cholesterol, and improved glycaemic control in type 2 diabetes.[17] Serious adverse effects include a rise in blood pressure and pulmonary hypertension. Less serious side-effects include headache, dry mouth, anorexia, constipation, insomnia, rhinitis, and pharyngitis in up to 30% of people taking sibutramine.[13]

Box 4.4: Monitoring treatment for sibutramine
- Monitor pulse and blood pressure every two weeks for three months then monthly until six months. Keep monitoring regularly thereafter.
- Monitor for signs of pulmonary hypertension.
- Encourage healthy sensible eating patterns and increased regular exercise.
- Weigh at each review attendance.
- Start on 10 mg once daily.
- If weight loss is less than 2 kg after four weeks, increase to 15 mg per day.
- Then, if weight loss is less than 2 kg over a four week period on the higher dose, discontinue.
- The maximum period of treatment is one year.

Screening Mrs Hart for depression and anxiety may be worthwhile, as psychological factors have been shown to be major predictors of weight gain in middle-aged women.[18]

Reducing dietary fat

Mrs Hart claimed that she already minimises fat in her diet. Less total fat or less of any individual fatty acid fraction in the diet is beneficial. A reduction of over 20% in total serum cholesterol concentration can result in a corresponding 25% fall in mortality from coronary heart disease.[6]

A recent systematic review of trials of diets that modified or reduced fat intake for at least six months has concluded that there is a:

> small but potentially important reduction in cardiovascular risk with reduction or modification of dietary fat intake, seen particularly in trials of longer duration.[19]

There were reductions in cardiovascular events of up to 24% in trials lasting for at least two years. But it was not clear whether it was the duration of the intervention or the length of follow up that was critical in determining whether the intervention was effective. There was little effect on total mortality.[19]

Physical activity

Mrs Hart may not be sure what type of physical activity she could try if she has led a sedentary life recently. Tell her that good advice is to:

> try to build up gradually to take half an hour of moderate intensity physical activity on five or more days of the week. Activities like brisk walking, cycling, swimming, dancing and gardening are good options.[20]

Warn Mrs Hart that physical inactivity doubles the risk of coronary heart disease, is a major risk factor for stroke and contributes to the increased frequency of overweight and obesity. There is a graded inverse relationship between physical activity and the risk of coronary events occurring.

In the general UK population, only a third of men (33%) and a fifth of women (21%) meet the current guidelines for physical activity – of moderate or vigorous activity for at least 30 minutes at a time, on five or more days a week.

Alcohol

Alcohol has nearly as much energy as fat at 7 kcal/g. It can compromise a weight-reducing diet, providing hidden calories. It is thought to alter the pattern of fat distribution encouraging a 'beer belly'. Excessive amounts of alcohol act as a central depressant and sap initiative and will power, reducing enthusiasm for physical exercise. Mrs Hart has already admitted to drinking excessive alcohol – a half to full bottle of wine per day, which probably add up to an average four or five units of alcohol per day and more than 30 units per week. The government recommends that women should drink no more than two to three units of alcohol per day and men three to four units per day, as women are more sensitive to the adverse effects of alcohol than men.[21]

It is widely believed that drinking red wine is good for the heart, but this benefit applies only to those groups at risk of coronary heart disease – men over 40 years and post-menopausal women – and is at its greatest benefit between one and two units of alcohol per day (all forms of alcohol and not just red wine).[21]

Around one-fifth of adults attending primary care are heavy drinkers – their drinking is generally missed by their GPs even though problem drinkers consult their GPs twice as often as other patients.[22] People do not usually seek help for their alcohol problems directly but present with other complaints such as dyspepsia, sleeplessness, heart arrhythmias or psychosocial problems. Early detection of and counselling in alcohol misuse, by primary care doctors as a brief alcohol intervention, is known to be effective but many GPs seem to consider that the drinking of alcohol is part of a patient's private life that should not be invaded if it is not presented as a problem.[23,24]

The simplest way to detect heavy drinking is to ask the person about their alcohol consumption – how much and how often. You could use the CAGE questionnaire where two or more positive answers suggest that the patient has a problem with alcohol:

* have you ever felt you ought to **C**ut down on your drinking?
* have people **A**nnoyed you by criticising your drinking?
* have you ever felt bad or **G**uilty about your drinking?
* have you ever had a drink first thing in the morning (**E**ye-opener) to steady your nerves or get rid of a hangover?

A good approach to take with Mrs Hart will be to spend five minutes with her now or at another appointment discussing the costs, risks and benefits from her perspective. Emphasise that she needs to reduce or stop her alcohol intake. Discuss with her what further support the practice or other agencies can offer.[25] Although there is no reliable laboratory marker for the effects of excessive alcohol consumption, you could arrange blood tests to see if the mean corpuscular volume is raised or liver function tests are abnormal – an isolated or disproportionately high gamma glutamyl transpeptidase (GGT) may be due to liver enzyme induction caused by alcohol, but could also be caused by other drugs such as phenytoin.

Sexual health and cervical screening

The practice nurse will be happy to review Mrs Hart's sexual health at her well woman check. A sexual health history fits in well with general enquiries during the check. She would not, of course, fall into the trap of making assumptions from Mrs Hart's appearance that she is, or has not been, exposed to sexual health risks! She will need to enquire about whether Mrs Hart has a current partner, if she is sexually active with this partner, and how long she has been with this partner. This can lead into a past history of changes of partnerships to give an estimation of her risk of acquiring sexually transmitted infections. Remember not to make assumptions that a patient is with a partner currently, or that any partnership is heterosexual.

Approximately 3000 new cases of cervical cancer are diagnosed each year in England and Wales, leading to about 1200 deaths.[26] About half of the women who present with late stage cervical cancer have never had a cervical smear. The presence of human papilloma virus (HPV) types 16 and 18 (and less commonly some of the other types of HPV) has been shown to be associated with the development of cervical cancer. The risk of acquiring HPV increases with having larger numbers of sexual partners, or a partner who has had many previous sexual partners.

The current cervical screening test is based on taking a sample of cells from the cervix with a wooden or plastic shaped spatula. The material collected is spread on a glass slide and sprayed with fixative. Specially trained cytologists examine the slide for abnormal cells. Relatively high numbers of slides are inadequate for examination because the cells are obscured by debris or blood, or are too thick or thin. Fatigue by cytologists is a significant cause of failure to avoid false-negative or false-positive results. The newer liquid-based cytology has a much lower rate of inadequate slides and clearer, more easily read, slides with the potential for automated slide examination. The sample is collected from the cervix in the same way, but using a special plastic broom-like device which is swept over the transitional zone five times to collect cellular material. The broom is rinsed in a vial of preservative. The vial is mixed in the laboratory and treated by an automated process to remove unwanted material. The remaining suspension of cells can be stained and the prepared slide looks much clearer for examination. The automation of the slide examination is also under trial. The proportion of inadequate smears (and subsequent repeat tests required) is greatly reduced.[27]

You or the practice nurse might need to explain to Mrs Hart that cervical screening at between three and five year intervals provides the best chance of picking up abnormal cells. Decreasing the interval to less than three years increases the pick-up rate only slightly in those with a previous negative test. Most authorities suggest that screening should be every three years initially until two or three negative results have been obtained, then five yearly.

Recommendations that are in the process of evaluation are to start screening at three-yearly intervals from the age of 25 years, and to switch to five-yearly intervals after the age of 49 years, discontinuing screening at 64 years of age in people who have had negative tests.[28]

Box 4.5:   Case study continued

Mrs Hart is not sure that she can give up smoking while she still feels so distressed over her friend's heart attack, but decides to go to the local leisure centre to enrol on an exercise programme. When she attends for her routine cervical smear, she tells the practice nurse that the regular exercise helps to relax her so that she drinks less and she has started to reduce her smoking as well.

Collecting data to demonstrate your learning, competence, performance and standards of service delivery: women's health

Example cycle of evidence 4.1

- Focus: clinical care
- Other relevant focus of evidence: smoking cessation

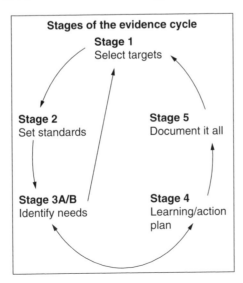

Stages of the evidence cycle

Stage 1 Select targets

Stage 2 Set standards

Stage 5 Document it all

Stage 3A/B Identify needs

Stage 4 Learning/action plan

Box 4.6:   Case study

Miss Flower has just had her first baby. At five pounds the baby was small for a full-term baby. Miss Flower is a smoker and she tells you that apart from the midwife mentioning that she should stop smoking when she first booked in for her pregnancy, no one else in the practice has ever advised her to stop smoking in the past when she has come for contraceptive or other healthcare.

This is just an example. Keep your task simple. You could choose three or four cycles of evidence to demonstrate your competence each year.

Stage 1: Select your aspirations for good practice

The excellent GP has:

- a structured approach for managing long-term health problems and preventive care.

Stage 2: Set the standards for your outcomes

Outcomes might include:

- the way learning is applied
- a learnt skill
- a protocol
- a strategy that is implemented
- meeting recommended standards.

- Every patient attending for antenatal care in first trimester or for contraceptive care is asked if they smoke and has their smoking history recorded.
- All pregnant women who smoke are offered advice about the risks of smoking and the benefits of quitting and further support and help.

Stage 3A: Identify your learning needs

- Self-assess your knowledge of the magnitude and nature of health risks associated with women who are smokers and especially those who are pregnant.

- Carry out a patient survey: ask ten consecutive patients who smoke (some should be pregnant) if they have received advice about smoking within the previous two years, and if so, how appropriate the advice was perceived to be, when it had been given and by whom.

Stage 3B: Identify your service needs

Any of the needs assessment exercises in 3A may also reveal service needs.

- Audit the smoking status of patients attending antenatal care in the last trimester for: existence of record of smoking status, extent of advice and support or help offered, and the change of smoking behaviour at the postnatal appointment.
- Carry out a significant event audit of cases of babies born to mothers who smoke who have health problems that might be associated with mother's smoking status, e.g. low birth weight, ear and chest infections in the first 12 months.

Stage 4: Make and carry out a learning and action plan

- Read up about risks of smoking and provision of best practice in motivating people to stop smoking.
- Talk to smokers at an informal group, e.g. in the waiting room during antenatal clinic, and actively listen to their feedback about improving services and the quality and extent of the advice they have received about stopping smoking.
- Audiotape (with patient's informed consent) a consultation (or two) where you give advice to a patient who is a smoker, offer them further help and try to motivate them to stop. Ask a health promotion expert to comment on your approach and give targeted feedback to you about your knowledge, skills and attitudes.

Stage 5: Document your learning, competence, performance and standards of service delivery

- Conduct patient surveys of smokers – two separate cohorts of patients at different time periods before and after putting your learning and action plan into practice, or one cohort of the same patients surveyed twice over time.
- Develop a practice protocol relating to smoking cessation.

- Carry out a re-audit of recording in antenatal patients' notes of smoking status, extent of advice and support or help offered, and the change of smoking behaviour at follow up.

Box 4.7:   Case study continued

Miss Flower's baby thrives as she makes up her mind not to inflict passive smoking on her baby or her partner at home. She quits after only using nicotine replacement therapy for a month and has not resumed smoking 12 months later.

Example cycle of evidence 4.2

- Focus: probity
- Other relevant focus of evidence: smoking cessation

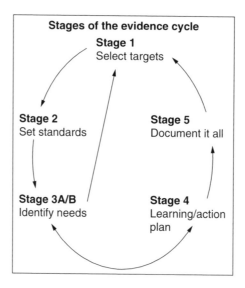

Stages of the evidence cycle

Stage 1
Select targets

Stage 2
Set standards

Stage 5
Document it all

Stage 3A/B
Identify needs

Stage 4
Learning/action plan

Box 4.8:   Case study

Dr Card, the practice GP lead for coronary heart disease, decided to work with the practice manager to tighten up the practice structure for delegating responsibility and delivering care. In an external inspection by the Commission for Health Improvement (CHI), the reviewers had noted that patient-identifiable information about smoking cessation was being passed to the PCO to trigger payments to practices without proper accountability. Dr Card aimed to clarify the team's roles and responsibilities for smoking cessation in such a way that the outcomes could be generalised to other areas of the practice.

This is just an example. Keep your task simple. You could choose three or four cycles of evidence to demonstrate your competence each year.

Stage 1: Select your aspirations for good practice

The excellent GP:

- ensures that his or her financial affairs are capable of withstanding searching outside audit
- has effective systems in the practice so that all team members understand their personal and collective responsibilities for the care and safety of patients.

Stage 2: Set the standards for your outcomes

Outcomes might include:

- the way learning is applied
- a learnt skill
- a protocol
- a strategy that is implemented
- meeting recommended standards.

- Compose and agree standards and processes for the way in which practice team members take responsibility for offering, providing and claiming for undertaking smoking cessation services.

Stage 3A: Identify your learning needs

- Reflect on how lines of responsibility work in the practice team, including how sure you are about who should do what and who takes responsibility for opportunistic and systematic advice to patients who smoke.
- Prepare for, and run, a tutorial for the GP registrar on probity about making claims for payments from the PCO. Self-assess your ability to answer his/her questions and challenges.

Stage 3B: Identify your service needs

> Any of the needs assessment exercises in 3A may also reveal service needs.

- Review the practice protocols for line management and accountability with the practice team in respect of all aspects of smoking cessation services. You should look for gaps and inconsistencies and include staff knowledge and skills, resources and promotional literature, finance claims and complaints.

Stage 4: Make and carry out a learning and action plan

- Attend relevant clinical management workshops.
- Update the practice protocol for smoking cessation to address gaps and inconsistencies identified in section 3B. Discuss at practice team meeting.
- Read the job evaluation handbook to understand what levels of knowledge and skills and other qualities practice team members should have.[29]

Stage 5: Document your learning, competence, performance and standards of service delivery

- Develop revised practice protocols about the lines of responsibility.
- Develop revised job descriptions of staff to reflect enhanced responsibilities.
- Keep a record of claims for undertaking smoking cessation services – with no patient-identifiable information.

Box 4.9:   Case study continued

Once Dr Card completed the exercise, he audited how all the clinical and non-clinical members of the practice team used the revised practice protocol for managing smoking cessation. The practice manager verified that the practice was not making false claims for providing smoking cessation services or missing out on payments. Dr Card worked with the practice manager to look at how the updated protocol could be generalised to provision of other enhanced services.

Example cycle of evidence 4.3

- Focus: maintaining good medical practice
- Other relevant focus of evidence: management of obesity

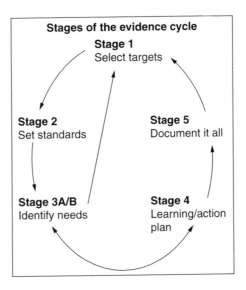

Box 4.10:   Case study

When Mrs Chubb got promotion she found that she was nervous about giving talks to groups of people and realised that her self-confidence was undermined by her obesity. After trying to lose weight herself with some success, she has come to you for a prescription for the slimming tablets she has heard about from her friend.

This is just an example. Keep your task simple. You could choose three or four cycles of evidence to demonstrate your competence each year.

Stage 1: Select your aspirations for good practice

The excellent GP:

- is up to date with developments in clinical practice and regularly reviews his or her knowledge and performance.

Stage 2: Set the standards for your outcomes

Outcomes might include:

- the way learning is applied
- a learnt skill
- a protocol
- a strategy that is implemented
- meeting recommended standards.

- Audit of your prescribing of anti-obesity medications shows that your clinical performance is in line with NICE guidance.
- Audit of patients for whom you have prescribed anti-obesity drugs demonstrates weight loss.

Stage 3A: Identify your learning needs

- Record in your reflective diary entries about overweight or obese patients requesting anti-obesity drugs. Consider how sure you are about the NICE guidelines about which patients may receive orlistat or sibutramine.
- Survey ten consecutive patients whom you have advised about their weight. Ask them if they consider that you are good at explaining options and best practice to them as patients.
- Record unsolicited or requested comments from the rest of the practice team about your management of patients with obesity.

Stage 3B: Identify your service needs

Any of the needs assessment exercises in 3A may also reveal service needs.

- Compare your own prescribing practice with that of others in the practice team and against NICE guidance.

- Record how the practice team deals with protests or other negative comments from patients denied anti-obesity drugs. This should be because they are outside NICE guidelines e.g. their BMI is too low, they have lost too little weight to justify starting an anti-obesity drug or the time limit for pre-scribing has expired.
- Organise or delegate organisation of a patient survey to the practice manager, which includes obese patients, enquiring about the quality of information given by the practice team, or local health promotion staff, about weight management.

Stage 4: Make and carry out a learning and action plan

- Download and read NICE guidance relating to the prescribing of anti-obesity drugs.
- Talk to obese patients and listen to their perspectives about adverse effects/benefits of anti-obesity drugs.
- Compose practice protocol as part of an in-house educational meeting.
- Audit the change in weight of overweight/obese patients over a 12 month period, whether or not they have received anti-obesity drugs. Flag their notes on computer screens so that successive GPs and practice nurses monitor their weight.

Stage 5: Document your learning, competence, performance and standards of service delivery

- Keep written reflections on your gain in knowledge and skills.
- Conduct a re-audit of treatment of obese patients against NICE guidance and the practice protocol (enclose revised protocol).
- Record the findings of the patient survey, including obese patients, about the quality of information given about weight management.

Box 4.11:   Case study continued

Mrs Chubb did receive orlistat because the course of medication was justified according to NICE criteria. She managed to lose two stone in weight over the following 12 months and started to regain the weight in the first six months off orlistat.

Example cycle of evidence 4.4

- Focus: maintaining good medical practice
- Other relevant focus of evidence: managing patients who drink excessive alcohol

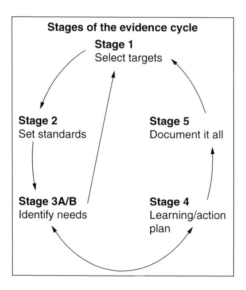

Stages of the evidence cycle

Stage 1 — Select targets

Stage 2 — Set standards

Stage 3A/B — Identify needs

Stage 4 — Learning/action plan

Stage 5 — Document it all

Box 4.12:   Case study

Mrs Mellow has been coming to see you and others in the practice frequently over the past year with minor complaints such as dyspepsia, irritability and difficulties getting to sleep. She complains about having to walk to the surgery to see you because she's lost her driving licence after a drink-driving offence. The penny drops about her heavy drinking being the likely cause of many of her symptoms! You determine to be more alert to hidden problems with alcohol in future.

This is just an example. Keep your task simple. You could choose three or four cycles of evidence to demonstrate your competence each year.

Stage 1: Select your aspirations for good practice

The excellent GP:

- makes sound management decisions, which are based on good practice and evidence.

Stage 2: Set the standards for your outcomes

Outcomes might include:

- the way learning is applied
- a learnt skill
- a protocol
- a strategy that is implemented
- meeting recommended standards.

- You and members of the primary care team are skilled in the recognition and management of people who drink excessive alcohol.

Stage 3A: Identify your learning needs

- Ask patients to complete an exit questionnaire about their lifestyle habits as they leave having consulted you. They can complete it in the surgery and leave it in a secure collection box at reception. Compare this with the records about smoking, alcohol and exercise habits in their medical notes.
- Write down the four questions from the CAGE questionnaire and check to see if you have remembered them correctly so that you can pose them to patients (*see* page 71).

Stage 3B: Identify your service needs

Any of the needs assessment exercises in 3A may also reveal service needs.

- Conduct a SCOT (strengths, challenges, opportunities and threats) analysis of recognition and management of patients who have excessive alcohol intake. You might discuss this with the practice team over a focused coffee break or as part of another meeting.
- Visit a neighbouring practice known for the well co-ordinated way they manage lifestyle screening and preventive care of those with problems

from heavy drinking, from the time patients present to the reception desk to when they leave the consulting room.

- Review your patient literature relating to limits on alcohol consumption to see if it is in date and appropriate for your patient population.
- Discuss the modes of effective communication to patients and staff about alcohol intake within the practice team at a practice meeting or with an adviser from the primary care organisation.
- Undertake a training needs analysis for you and the practice team. Ascertain any gaps between expected and actual levels of knowledge and skills in relation to recognising and managing patients who are heavy drinkers of alcohol.

Stage 4: Make and carry out a learning and action plan

- Organise a 'how to do it' workshop on the national recommendations for alcohol intake and the carrying out of brief interventions in primary care. Ask a health promotion expert to run it as an in-house event for all the practice team.
- Write a short newsletter for patients describing lifestyle interventions (including alcohol) available at the practice and through other agencies.
- Plan to address challenges and opportunities that have emerged from the SCOT analysis. Make changes such as to the way care is delivered or how information about alcohol is recorded or how the team communicates.

Stage 5: Document your learning, competence, performance and standards of service delivery

- Conduct a training needs analysis of you and the practice team in relation to section 3B above.
- Produce a personal development plan recording the gaps in your knowledge and skills and completion of your learning plan.
- Keep records of the SCOT analysis and the plan to address challenges and opportunities in relation to recognition and management of patients (and staff) with alcohol problems.

Box 4.13:   Case study continued

Mrs Mellow's son is home from university and comes to see you complaining of dyspepsia, irritability and difficulties with sleep. You ask him about his lifestyle and smoking and drinking habits. You pose the four questions in the CAGE questionnaire. He is surprised that you think his regular intake of three or four pints of beer a day might be the cause of his complaints as he feels he drinks a lot less than his mates. He agrees to reduce his drinking for a trial period and to come and see you again in a few weeks' time.

Example cycle of evidence 4.5

- Focus: relationships with patients
- Other relevant focus of evidence: health promotion by yourself and the practice team

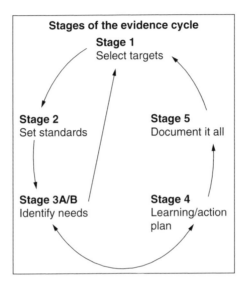

Stages of the evidence cycle

Stage 1
Select targets

Stage 2
Set standards

Stage 5
Document it all

Stage 3A/B
Identify needs

Stage 4
Learning/action plan

Box 4.14: Case study

As Mrs Test neared her 50th birthday she wanted a full 'MOT' to check that she had no health problems. So she contacted the surgery to see if she could book in for a well woman check. She explained that she just wanted a mammogram and blood tests. She added that she could do without the lecture she knew she would get about smoking and lack of exercise.

This is just an example. Keep your task simple. You could choose three or four cycles of evidence to demonstrate your competence each year.

Stage 1: Select your aspirations for good practice

The excellent GP:

- gives patients the information they need about their problem in a way they can understand
- respects the right of patients to refuse treatments or tests.

Stage 2: Set the standards for your outcomes

Outcomes might include:

- the way learning is applied
- a learnt skill
- a protocol
- a strategy that is implemented
- meeting recommended standards.

- Produce an up-to-date protocol for a well woman clinic individualised for age groups of women.
- Keep a bank of health promotion literature and other resources linked to the processes undertaken in a well woman clinic.

Stage 3A: Identify your learning needs

- Issue anonymised comment slips to the next ten consecutive female patients who attend the well woman clinic or who book in for a health promotion check with you or the practice nurse.
- Ensure that you and the reception and nursing staff keep notes of direct feedback from individual patients about any aspect of health promotion of lifestyle advice and look for trends or patterns.
- Consider if you are competent to give patients up-to-date information and balanced advice about the risks and benefits of screening. For example, breast screening for women in their 40s, bone density scanning for those with a family history of osteoporosis, or cervical cytology for those in their late 50s who have always had normal cervical smears.

Stage 3B: Identify your service needs

Any of the needs assessment exercises in 3A may also reveal service needs.

- Compare the views of different types of patients, if it is clear from the comment slips (as in section 3A) that they are different, e.g. women living in inner cities or in rural communities, or women in employment or not employed, or by socio-economic characteristics as appropriate.
- Undertake a significant event audit with key members of the practice team of e.g. a woman who presents with a stroke in her late 50s and who has never had her blood pressure recorded in her notes.
- Audiotape (with patients' informed consent) you and the practice nurse giving health promotion advice. Swap tapes and peer review for style of communication and content.

Stage 4: Make and carry out a learning and action plan

- Attend an update lecture on screening and ask the experts questions about risks and benefits of screening as posed in section 3A. Write down answers to study and reflect on later.
- Study the feedback from patients and reflect on how to make changes to meet the needs of patients more effectively. Revise the protocol for the well woman clinic accordingly in discussion with the practice team.
- Read the manufacturers' literature that patients receive with nicotine replacement and anti-obesity therapy and other health promotion literature you have been distributing to patients, so that you know what information patients may be reading.

Stage 5: Document your learning, competence, performance and standards of service delivery

- Write a list of the frequently asked questions from patients and the answers, and make it available to practice nurses engaged in health promotion activities.
- Collect feedback from patients and the service improvement plan.
- Keep health promotion literature for patients that you have approved for distribution.
- Document a revised 'well woman check' protocol and the plans to monitor your/colleagues' adherence to protocol.
- Peer review reports of audiotaped consultations.

Box 4.15:   Case study continued

Mrs Test attends for a well person check with the practice nurse. The nurse is flexible and agrees with a laugh that she will not give Mrs Test a lecture on her bad habits, but offers help in the future if Mrs Test feels she could do with it.

References

1 Munafo M, Drury M, Wakley G, Chambers R and Murphy M (2003) *Smoking Cessation Matters in Primary Care.* Radcliffe Medical Press, Oxford.

2 Prochaska JO, DiClemente CC and Norcross JC (1992) In search of how people change. Applications to addictive behaviours. *Am Psychol.* **47**: 1102–14.

3 Riemsma RP, Pattenden J, Bridle C *et al.* (2003) Systematic review of the effectiveness of stage based interventions to promote smoking cessation. *BMJ.* **326**: 1175–7.

4 Chambers R and Wakley G (2002) *Obesity and Overweight Matters in Primary Care.* Radcliffe Medical Press, Oxford.

5 World Health Organization (1997) *Obesity: preventing and managing the global epidemic.* World Health Organization, Geneva.

6 National Audit Office (2001) *Tackling Obesity in England.* National Audit Office, London.

7 Garrow J and Summerbell C (2002) Obesity. In: Department of Health. *Health Needs Assessment.* Radcliffe Medical Press, Oxford.

8 Stevens V, Obarzanek E, Cook N *et al.* (2001) Long-term weight loss and changes in blood pressure: results of the trials of hypertension prevention, Phase 11. *Ann Intern Med.* **134**: 1–11.

9 Maryon Davis A, Giles A and Rona R (2000) *Tackling Obesity: a toolbox for local partnership action.* Faculty of Public Health, Royal College of Physicians of the UK, London.

10 Bravata DM, Sanders L, Huang J *et al.* (2003) Efficacy and safety of low-carbohydrate diets. *JAMA.* **289(14)**: 1837–49.

11 Moore A and McQuay H (eds) (2003) Low carbohydrate diets – two RCTs and a systematic review. *Bandolier 113.* **10(2)**: 4–5.

12 Joint Formulary Committee (2003) *British National Formulary.* British Medical Association and Royal Pharmaceutical Society of Great Britain, London.

13 Godlee F (ed.) (2003) *Clinical Evidence.* Issue 9. BMJ Publishing Group, London.

14 National Institute for Clinical Excellence (2001) *Guidance on the Use of Orlistat for the Treatment of Obesity in Adults.* NICE, London.

15 National Institute for Clinical Excellence (2001) *Guidance on the Use of Sibutramine for the Treatment of Obesity in Adults.* NICE, London.

16 Apfelbaum M, Vague P, Ziegler O *et al.* (1999) Long-term maintenance of weight loss after a very low calorie diet: a randomised trial of the efficacy and tolerability of sibutramine. *Am J Med.* **106**: 179–84.

17 Sjostrum L, Rissanen A, Andersen T *et al.* for the European Multicentre Orlistat Study Group (2000) Randomized double blind placebo controlled multicenter study of sibutramine in obese hypertensive patients. *Cardiology.* **94**: 152–8.

18   Sammel MD, Grisso JA, Freeman EW *et al.* (2003) Weight gain among women in the late reproductive years. *Fam Pract.* **20**: 401–9.

19   Hooper L, Summerbell C, Higgins J *et al.* (2001) Dietary fat intake and prevention of cardiovascular disease: systematic review. *BMJ.* **322**: 757–63.

20   Health Education Authority (1998) *Managing Weight. A workbook for health and other professionals.* Health Education Authority, London.

21   www.alcoholconcern.org.uk.

22   Kaner EF, Healther N, Brodie J *et al.* (2001) Patient and practitioner characteristics predict brief alcohol intervention in primary care. *Br J Gen Pract.* **471**: 822–7.

23   Anderson P (1993) Effectiveness of general practice interventions for patients with harmful alcohol consumption. *Br J Gen Pract.* **43**: 386–9.

24   Aira M, Kauhanen J, Larivaara P and Rautio P (2003) Factors influencing inquiry about patients' alcohol consumption by primary health care physicians: qualitative semi-structured interview study. *Fam Pract.* **20**: 270–5.

25   World Health Organization (2000) Diagnosis and management of alcohol misuse in primary care. Reproduced in *Guidelines.* **20**: 153–5.

26   Department of Health (1999) *Bulletin on Cervical Screening Programme: England 1998–9.* Department of Health, London. Also available from www.doh.gov.uk/public/sb9932.htm and www.cancerscreening.nhs.uk/cervical.

27   National Institute for Clinical Excellence (2003) *Final Appraisal Determination – guidance on the use of liquid-based cytology for cervical screening.* Review of existing guidance number 5. http://www.nice.org.uk/pdf/FAD_LBC.pdf.

28   Sasieni P, Adams J and Cusik J (2003) Benefits of cervical screening at different ages: evidence from the UK audit of screening histories. *Br J Cancer.* **89(1)**: 88–93.

29   Department of Health (2003) *Job Evaluation Handbook.* Version 1. Department of Health, London.

5

Contraception

Box 5.1: Case study

Two young women attend the practice together. Miss Brain explains that she is registered at your practice and has brought Miss Giddy to see you so that she can go on the pill. Miss Giddy will not go to see her own doctor at another practice because 'He'll just give me a lecture'.

What issues you should cover

Seeing patients for contraception-only services and confidentiality

Explain to Miss Giddy that she can be seen for contraception-only services without being registered for general medical services. What she says to this doctor is kept confidential. That is, no one else needs to know unless there is a risk to her health or to someone else's health, which would mean that other people would need to know. It would always be discussed with her if confidential information needed to be passed to someone else. You would like to let her regular doctor know about the contraceptive consultation but only if she agrees. Give her the choice of being seen by herself or with her friend.

Risk of pregnancy

Explain that you need to know a bit about her to find out if it is safe for her to start taking the contraceptive pill. First, establish if she is already sexually active. If she is, then you need to know if she is using any other method of contraception (e.g. condoms). Ask if, and when, she has had any unprotected sexual intercourse and the date of her last menstrual period, in case she needs emergency contraception or is already pregnant (*see* information on emergency contraception later in this chapter).

If she has not started having sexual intercourse, explain that although lots of young people pretend to be having sexual intercourse, confidential surveys have shown that eight out of ten young people under the age of 16 years have not actually started having sexual intercourse. It may be better for her to go on the pill just in case but she does not have to have sexual intercourse unless she wants to.

Age and the law

You may not be given correct information about her date of birth (or her identity) if she is fearful that she will not be given contraceptive advice because she is under 16 years of age. If she is living in the parental home, whatever her age, it is much simpler for her to have discussed her need for contraception at home so that there is no need for concealment. Discuss how she might do this, if she has not already done so. The younger the woman, the more important it is to establish whether this discussion has taken place and whether the woman herself understands the full implications of her actions. Keep in mind the Fraser Guidelines (*see* Chapter 3).

Her plans for the future

Find out how important it is for her not to be pregnant. She may say that she is not bothered whether she gets pregnant or not. This is often because she has no belief in her own ability to control her future – or because she does not have any vision of her future at all; things just happen to her. Talking to her about what she wants to do in the future can help her to see when a pregnancy might be more easily managed.

It may be extremely important for her not to become pregnant. Women who have definite plans – for a job, for training or further education – are usually well motivated to use contraception. Some young women are definite (at least for the time being) that they never want children.

Reasons why she may not have used contraception

The Social Exclusion Unit report[1] attributes high rates of teenage conception in the UK to young people's:

- low expectations
- lack of knowledge about contraception and how it can be obtained
- lack of understanding about what is involved in forming relationships and parenting

- reception of mixed messages from society – 'it sometimes seems as if sex is compulsory but contraception is illegal' as one of the young people cited in the report said.

In a national survey of 515 teenagers aged 12 to 17 years old, more than half of the respondents said that the main reason young people do not use birth control was because of drinking alcohol or using drugs. Boys and girls gave similar answers. Half of the teenagers quizzed thought another common reason for young people having unprotected sex was pressure from partners who do not want to use contraception. Young adolescents aged 12 to 14 years old were as likely as the older teenagers to say this.[2]

Problems associated with teenage pregnancy

The death rate for babies of teenage mothers is 60% higher than that for babies of older mothers and maternal and fetal risks are highest in under-16 year olds.

Pregnant teenagers are more likely than mothers aged 20 to 35 years to have low income, poor education, be unwed, be cigarette smokers, and have poor nutrition. The Acheson report on health inequalities recognised that teenage mothers and their children are at higher risk of experiencing adverse health, educational, social and economic outcomes, compared to older mothers and their children.[3]

Teenage pregnancy is a cause and effect of inequalities in health. Teenage mothers tend to have poor antenatal care, low birth weight infants and higher infant mortality rates. Teenage parents tend to miss out on education and have substantially lower incomes. They are more likely to suffer from postnatal depression and relationship breakdown.

Box 5.2:   Risk factors for teenage pregnancy[2]

- Having a teenage mother
- Divorced parents
- Deprivation
- Being a child living in care
- Educational problems
- Sexual abuse
- Ethnicity
- Mental health problems
- Crime

What she may know about contraception already

Some young women are well informed and have read many leaflets. Others know little or nothing. Make sure that you mention other methods of contraception apart from the pill that her friend has already suggested. Using a leaflet that summarises all the methods enables you to go through each method and its level of contraceptive protection quite rapidly, so that she can make her own choice for discussion in more detail.[4]

Check that she is safe to use her chosen contraceptive

Most young women will be healthy and have no contraindications to any method of contraception. For them, any method of contraception is preferable to the risks of pregnancy (although you can tell her that abstinence is the safest method of all, provided it does not fail!). You need to take a medical history to ensure that her chosen method will not do harm. Checking her blood pressure before giving contraceptives containing oestrogen is essential, but other physical examination is not necessary unless indicated by the history. Obesity and/or smoking increase her risks of venous thrombosis and cardiovascular disease. The absolute risk of venous thrombosis in a young woman is small, but lifestyle advice now may help her to make changes to avoid an increased risk in the future. However, keep in mind that she has come for contraceptive advice, not a lecture on her bad habits – or she will not want to return to see you.

You may wish to use a checklist to exclude contraindications. The World Health Organization (WHO) publishes a checklist with advice on cautions and contraindications.[5] A UK adaptation of the WHO advice appears on the website for the Faculty of Family Planning and Reproductive Health Care.[6]

Summarising where the consultation has reached

The consultation has probably already lasted ten minutes. You may need to summarise where you are and ask her what she wants to do next. If she has an urgent need for contraception (most young people do not attend until they do need it urgently) your next action is to take the extra time to help her learn how to use the method she has chosen. If she wants to use a long-acting method, she might be better using a short-acting method temporarily and returning later. This gives both of you time to discuss the method in more depth and for a more considered decision on a method that she cannot change easily. (Long-acting methods are discussed later in this chapter in Table 5.1.)

She and her sexual partner should use condoms for protection against method failure (common when people first start using contraception) and against sexually transmitted infections (STIs). She should be clear that most people do not have any symptoms from STIs and that appearances are no guide as to whether someone is infected or not.

A young woman who is still living with her parents or guardians can be helped to realise that they may be worried about whether she is protected against pregnancy, but may be uncertain how to ask her if she is at risk. Talk about ways she might discuss this with them.

Using short-acting methods

Condoms

You may be able to supply condoms but, if not, you need to know how she can obtain them. If you supply them, show her how they are used and give her a leaflet for her partner. Discuss with her how she is going to ask her partner to use condoms, how she will carry condoms (many young people do not have handbags or pockets) and that the condom should be put on the penis after erection but before genital contact.

She can obtain free supplies from family planning clinics, sexual health clinics and youth clinics, such as Brook or locally developed services. You should know where the local suppliers are, when they are open, and how she can be seen (does she need an appointment or is it open access?). She can go with her sexual partner or he can obtain condoms from the same places himself, so that he can be sure how to use them correctly. She, or her partner, can buy condoms from many outlets, including vending machines, chemists, supermarkets and garages.

Female condoms (Femidom) need to be used carefully so that the penis is placed inside the polyurethane sleeve lining the vagina. They are rather expensive – but can be bought over the counter with no need for medical intervention. They are disliked by some people because of the 'plastic mac' feel and are noisy in use.

Oral methods

She may decide to start on the combined oral contraceptive (COC) or the progestogen-only pill (POP). It is useful to go through the leaflet with her that you will give her to take away.[4] This ensures that the advice you give and the advice in the leaflet are the same (or that you have hand-written any changes and explained the reasons for them). Tell her that the leaflet in the packet of pills may give slightly different advice depending on how long ago it was written.

Give her the choice of starting immediately or waiting for the first day of her next period. If she starts immediately, she should not rely on the pill for her contraception for the first seven days. If she starts on the first day of her menstrual cycle, she will be protected against pregnancy immediately, but will still need to use condoms for extra safety and protection against the risk of STIs.

Help her to decide what time of day will be easiest for her to remember to take her pill. Show her a packet of the pill she will be taking or a diagram in the leaflet of how to take the pill. Show her the section in the leaflet on what to do if she misses a pill and go through the instructions, as this is the commonest cause of failure. Advise her how to stop smoking if she is a cigarette smoker.

She should contact you or the practice nurse (explain how) or attend again before her review appointment if she has any queries that are not explained in the leaflet, or new serious health complaints. Point out the types of condition, listed in the leaflet, that should bring her to the doctor urgently (e.g. shortness of breath, leg pain and swelling, first or worsening migraine, or dizziness).

Emergency contraception[6–9]

One of the reasons Miss Giddy may be consulting you urgently rather than her own GP could be that she has had unprotected sexual intercourse and requires emergency contraception.

The oral emergency contraceptives, Levonelle or Levonelle-2, can be used up to 72 hours after unprotected intercourse, but the earlier the better. Levonelle and Levonelle-2 both contain the same doses of progestogen. Levonelle is the version bought over the counter and Levonelle-2 is the prescribed version. Levonelle is 95% effective in preventing pregnancy when taken within 24 hours of unprotected sexual intercourse. It is 85% effective when taken 25–48 hours later and only 58% effective when taken between 49 and 72 hours later.

Increased doses of hormone are necessary for patients on hepatic enzyme inducers such as phenytoin, carbamazepine or rifampicin to obtain the same blood levels. Most guidelines advise two pills followed by either another one or two 12 hours later.[6,7] Box 5.3 summarises the information you will need to elicit to decide whether oral emergency contraception should be prescribed and what advice to give. You could use this to draw up a practice protocol.

The insertion of a copper IUD up to five days after unprotected intercourse has an even lower failure rate (0.1%) than oral methods. It can be used up to five days after the calculated date of ovulation (i.e. the 19th day of a 28 day shortest cycle from the history, counting day 1 as the first day of bleeding) and successfully prevents implantation. The IUD can be removed at the next menstruation if it is not required or desired for continuing contraception.

Box 5.3: Emergency contraception tablets – basic information required and advice

Minimum information to be recorded in the notes prior to prescribing oral post-coital contraception should include:
- last menstrual period (LMP)
- cycle length
- date and time of unprotected sexual intercourse (UPSI)
- day of cycle of UPSI
- any other UPSI since LMP
- options discussed (oral/IUD)
- any interacting medication
- current liver disease.

Counselling should include:
- likelihood of nausea
- mode of action
- failure rate
- side-effects
- timing of next period
- action to take if next period is not on time
- discussion of future contraception needs.

Vomiting after taking emergency combined oral contraception
If the patient vomits within two hours of taking the pills, she should be advised to seek further medical advice. Domperidone 10 mg can be used to prevent vomiting.

Issuing guidelines
- Negotiate the time of the first and second doses and write them down.
- Go through the leaflet with the patient.
- Make follow-up arrangements or advise them to return one week after the expected date of the next period.
- Record whether emergency contraception was given or prescribed.

Remember that exposure to unprotected intercourse means exposure to possible sexual infection also, so informed consent for screening, especially for chlamydial infection, is usually required.

Long-acting contraception

Miss Giddy may wish to discuss her options if she wants to embark on long-acting contraception. If you have not got enough time to go through the alternatives in full detail you may supply her with leaflets or an audiotape about the possible types as shown in Table 5.1 and arrange to see her again

Table 5.1: Longer-acting methods of contraception

Method	For	Against
Injection Depo-Provera (medroxyprogesterone acetate) 150 mg given intramuscularly every 12 weeks or Noristerat (norethisterone oenanthate) 200 mg every 8 weeks	• Could be started with the next period or before if pregnancy can be excluded. • Effective after seven days, possibly sooner. • Lasts for 12 weeks (or 8 weeks for Noristerat), giving time to consider longer-term action. • Usually gives very light and infrequent periods or no bleeding at all. • Enhances breast milk flow. Is likely to give very light or absent menses once breast-feeding has stopped. • Very low failure rate.	• Weight gain common with Depo-Provera, less with Noristerat. • Has to return every 12 (or 8) weeks for another injection and may easily forget unless someone else takes the responsibility for reminding her. • Progestogenic side-effects may be unacceptable: acne, feeling constantly premenstrual, irregular or absent periods. • She may not have attained her peak bone mass because of her age, especially if she smokes or has a poor diet. Depo-Provera might increase the risk of a low bone mass. • Small theoretical risk to a breast-fed baby from the absorbed progestogen, especially if a baby is premature and has immature liver enzymes.
Implant (Implanon) Small plastic rod inserted in the bicipital groove of the upper arm releasing etonorgestrel over three years	• She would not require any other method for three years, giving time for reflection about her future needs. • If someone in the practice fits implants, she could have one fitted within five days of the start of her next period. • She does not have to remember anything for three years. • Very low failure rate.	• Usually cannot be done immediately and needs some time to set up a fitting. • If no one in practice fits these, patient may have to attend another venue. • Frequent spotting or light periods may not suit everyone and a few people have unacceptable progestogenic side-effects. • Recall system needed so that the implant is not forgotten.

continued opposite

Table 5.1: *continued*

Method	For	Against
Intrauterine device with copper (IUCD) Cu T380 Multiload 350 Nova-T380 Flexi-T	• Could be fitted immediately if facilities available and pregnancy can be excluded. • Would give protection for 5–10 years depending on device. • Cu T380 has a very low failure rate with the others only slightly higher. • Can be used as a post-coital method if she is at risk following unprotected intercourse.	• Might have to re-attend or attend a different venue if no facilities to fit it immediately. • Easier to fit in the multiparous uterus. • Success rates dependent more on the expertise of the person fitting it than on the type of device used. Health professionals who only fit a few devices each year have higher expulsion, bleeding, removal and perforation rates. • Usually increases the menstrual loss and may increase dysmenorrhoea if present. • Recall system needed so that it is not forgotten.
Intrauterine system with progesterone (IUS) Mirena	• Could be fitted within five days of the start of her next period if facilities are available. • Decreases menstrual loss, usually to none after first few months of irregular loss. • Would give protection for five years. • Failure rate is even lower than sterilisation.	• Might have to re-attend or attend a different venue if no facilities to fit it immediately. • Nulliparous women usually need cervical anaesthesia as the diameter of the device is wider than an IUD. • Success rates dependent more on the expertise of the person fitting it than on the type of device used. Specific training needed as different insertion technique to other IUCDs. • Decreases menstrual loss, usually to none after first few months of irregular loss. • Recall system needed so that it is not forgotten.

continued overleaf

Table 5.1:   *continued*

Method	For	Against
Female sterilisation	• Permanent and suitable for women who are certain they want no more children. • Low failure rate.	• Permanent and not suitable for anyone who is not certain or feels they will have lost their femininity. • Failure rate higher than vasectomy or IUS. • Usually requires referral to secondary care (long wait to be seen) and at least admission for day case surgery. Usually done under general anaesthesia with the attendant risks. • May require laparotomy if tubes cannot be visualised with the laparoscope. That would require a longer stay in hospital and longer recovery period.
Vasectomy	• Permanent and suitable for men who are certain they want no more children. • Low failure rate.	• Not suitable for anyone who is not certain about whether more children will ever be desired. • Usually done under local anaesthesia, occasionally under general with its attendant risks. • Temporary pain and discomfort in most men who can return to work after 48 hours. Manual workers require longer off work. • Some men develop epididymal cysts, or granulomas. Chronic pain develops in about 2% of men.

continued opposite

Table 5.1: *continued*

Method	For	Against
Combined contraceptive patch	• Only needs application weekly for three weeks, omitted for the fourth week. • Good cycle control. • Under the control of the woman if she wants to stop it at any time. • Low failure rate but not as low as any of the methods above.	• The oestrogen component can reduce breast milk flow. • The oestrogen component increases her thrombosis risk. • She has to remember it weekly. • It is expensive compared with the oral contraceptive pill.

soon. Don't forget to exclude pregnancy with a pregnancy test if necessary before starting her on a long-acting method. Provide the contraception at the right time of her menstrual cycle, for example you would give Depo-Provera, or insert an implant, within the first five days after her period has started.

Collecting data to demonstrate your learning, competence, performance and standards of service delivery: contraception

Example cycle of evidence 5.1

- Focus: clinical care
- Other relevant focus of evidence: probity

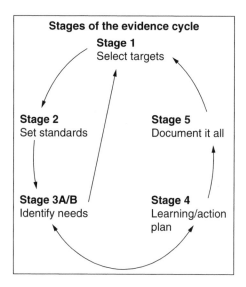

Stages of the evidence cycle

Stage 1
Select targets

Stage 2
Set standards

Stage 5
Document it all

Stage 3A/B
Identify needs

Stage 4
Learning/action plan

Box 5.4:   Case study

Miss Chance is a 15 year old who attends a Friday evening surgery to see the practice nurse on duty. The girl's mother is one of the morning receptionists at the surgery. This is the second week that this nurse has been working on her own in the treatment suite since starting work at the practice three months ago. The nurse contacts you to ask if she can give her some emergency contraceptive pills from the stock in the treatment room. The nurse has not done any family planning training but tells you she thinks she can go through the protocol she has been told is on the computer, if you would like her to try.

You have not previously assessed the competency of the practice nurse to do this task. It is not safe to assume that she will perform adequately, nor is it fair to give her this responsibility without training. She may be offering to do something outside her limits of competency because 'she does not know what she does not know'. She may also be pressurised by the patient for a quick solution because of the relationship with one of the receptionists. The patient should not receive inferior care just because she is the daughter of a member of staff.

This is just an example. Keep your task simple. You could choose three or four cycles of evidence to demonstrate your competence each year.

Stage 1: Select your aspirations for good practice

The excellent GP:

- responds rapidly to emergencies
- arranges appropriate training for practice staff in managing emergencies.

Stage 2: Set the standards for your outcomes

Outcomes might include:

- the way learning is applied
- a learnt skill
- a protocol
- a strategy that is implemented
- meeting recommended standards.

- Demonstrate consistent best practice in provision of emergency contraception to teenagers in respect of availability and accessibility and clinical management.
- Demonstrate best practice in the maintenance of confidentiality.
- Information about contraceptive services you provide is factual and verifiable, conforms with the law and with guidance issued by the Advertising Standards Authority e.g. in the practice leaflet.

- Information that you publish about the quality of your contraceptive services can be justified (e.g. that you do not claim that IUDs or vasectomies can be done at any time if patients have to make specific arrangements for that service).
- Information published about your services does not exploit patients' vulnerability or lack of medical knowledge or put pressure on people to use a service.

Stage 3A: Identify your learning needs

- Carry out with other practice staff a significant event audit e.g. a teenager who became pregnant after consulting you about contraception three months previously. This may throw up learning needs about emergency contraception (*see* Table 5.1 and Box 5.3) or about actively listening to patients.
- Record in your own reflective diary trends or comments relating to problems or issues of emergency contraception in teenagers. This might be to do with how well the services are running or about consultations with you or other GPs or nurses.
- Do a notes review to audit how often you discuss, and screen for, sexually transmitted infections. Exposure to unprotected intercourse is exposure to infection (unless within a monogamous partnership).
- Audit your own adherence to the practice protocol for emergency contraception.

Stage 3B: Identify your service needs

Any of the needs assessment exercises in 3A may also reveal service needs.

- Audit the accessibility of aspects of family planning services e.g. a patient survey to establish the interval between the time an appointment is requested by a teenager to making face-to-face contact with a nurse or GP. You may establish that this new practice nurse requires training in family planning to supplement the availability of your present staff, or that there are sufficient trained staff to cope with most of the demand.
- Observe the pathway of care received e.g. by a pregnant teenager who had presented to the reception desk at the GPs' surgery either before, or more than, 72 hours after unprotected sex.
- Check with staff that everyone is aware of the need for confidentiality, and how it should be maintained, e.g. the practice manager might use this case (anonymously) to illustrate the pitfalls and that no one should inadvertently mention seeing someone at the surgery.

- Ask the PCO or other external commentators to critique the information you supply about your contraceptive services (practice leaflet or other published information).

Stage 4: Make and carry out a learning and action plan

- Read up on latest recommendations for emergency contraception and revise the protocol if required.[6,7]
- Read up and discuss at a practice meeting the latest evidence about progestogen-only emergency contraception. You might want to be an innovator and extend the time limits for giving it from 72 hours to five days or modify the administration by giving both doses together.[10,11]
- Visit another practice where there is excellent practice in delivering appropriate care for teenagers and/or family planning services.

Stage 5: Document your learning, competence, performance and standards of service delivery

- Re-audit the consistent application of practice policy or protocol relating to emergency contraception.
- Repeat the teenage patient survey for timely access.
- Repeat your reflective diary.
- Audit the awareness of staff with a checklist about confidentiality.
- Produce a practice leaflet describing services provided in the practice.

Box 5.5:   Case study continued

You see Miss Chance yourself, and assess her need for emergency contraception. You should ensure that her confidentiality is assured. She is only just within the 72 hour limit for emergency contraception but does not want to have an IUD fitted. You give her both the Levonelle-2 pills immediately from your emergency stock (remembering to write the prescription to replace it). You discuss using continuing contraception, but she says she does not need it. You ask her to return to see you if she changes her mind and reassure her again about confidentiality. You discuss ways she might talk about her future needs for continuing contraception at home. You also give her a leaflet about the opening times and contact telephone numbers of the local clinics in case she would prefer to attend there. You remind the staff on duty about confidentiality.

Example cycle of evidence 5.2

- Focus: clinical care
- Other relevant focus of evidence: teaching and training

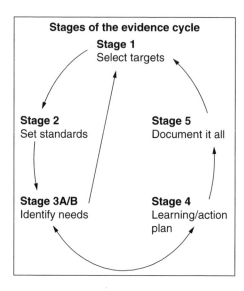

Stages of the evidence cycle

Stage 1
Select targets

Stage 2
Set standards

Stage 5
Document it all

Stage 3A/B
Identify needs

Stage 4
Learning/action plan

Box 5.6:　Case study

Mrs Daffy tells the GP registrar that her husband says she must be sterilised. She delivered her fifth child six weeks ago and has had two miscarriages as well. She has been prescribed some progestogen-only pills to start on the 21st day after delivery but says she has not had time to obtain them from the pharmacy yet. She adds that she doesn't like taking pills anyway. She is obviously overweight and from her medical record it can be seen that she is 29 years old, smokes but has normal blood pressure. She asks if it is okay to breast feed the baby who is crying loudly and two of her other children start investigating the drawers and cupboards in the consulting room. This is the first surgery session that the GP registrar has taken and he turns to you looking completely overwhelmed.

This is just an example. Keep your task simple. You could choose three or four cycles of evidence to demonstrate your competence each year.

Stage 1: Select your aspirations for good practice

The excellent GP:

- makes an adequate assessment of the patient's condition, based on the history and, if indicated, an appropriate examination
- provides or arranges investigations or treatment where necessary
- recognises and works within the limits of his/her competence and refers to another practitioner when indicated
- consults with colleagues and keep them informed when sharing the care of patients.

Stage 2: Set the standards for your outcomes

Outcomes might include:

- the way learning is applied
- a learnt skill
- a protocol
- a strategy that is implemented
- meeting recommended standards.

- Demonstrate consistent best practice in provision of continuing contraception to patients in respect of availability and accessibility and clinical management.
- Demonstrate best use of resources.
- Contribute to the education of students or colleagues willingly.
- Develop the skills, attitudes and practices of a competent teacher if you have responsibilities for teaching.
- Ensure that students and junior colleagues are properly supervised in line with the responsibilities you have for teaching them.

Stage 3A: Identify your learning needs

- Carry out a significant event audit with other practice staff e.g. looking at the reasons why Mrs Daffy or a similar patient had not used contraception previously. Had she defaulted from care or had there been failures in the system or standards of care?
- Examine a complaint e.g. about inadequate counselling before sterilisation or vasectomy. Do you need to use an up-to-date leaflet or a checklist to ensure that people have sufficient information to make an informed choice?

- Keep a reflective diary capturing trends or comments relating to problems or issues of longer-acting methods of contraception e.g. you might record that you no longer feel competent doing IUD or IUS fittings because of changes in devices and lack of practice due to low demand. You may want to provide implant fittings but lack the training.
- Ask for feedback from the GP registrar about the effectiveness of the supervision and whether he felt supported sufficiently during his steep learning curve in the realities of general practice contraception provision.

Stage 3B: Identify your service needs

> Any of the needs assessment exercises in 3A may also reveal service needs.

- Review the difficulty of finding the time to fit an IUD or IUS because of competing demands on your own time, or the practice nurse having insufficient time to prepare and assist with the procedure, or the non-availability of a suitable room in which to do the procedure.
- Perform a patient survey to ascertain the demand and when people would like to be able to access a service providing longer-acting methods.
- Audit the availability and adequacy of emergency resuscitation equipment and the training standards of health professionals to use it.
- Identify the registrar's learning style and what learning tasks you set to match his style.

Stage 4: Make and carry out a learning and action plan

- Attend a refresher course and practical training on modern IUD and IUS fitting. Learn how to fit and remove implants.
- Research the availability of provision of longer-acting methods of contraception and liaise with those services. Perhaps you might help to make a proposal to the PCO for more accessible local provision. This might involve finding out the comparative costs of various contraceptive options.
- Read up about alternative methods of contraception and the points to consider about sterilisation counselling.

Stage 5: Document your learning, competence, performance and standards of service delivery

- Retain any certificates of learning and competence achieved.
- Record and disseminate your learning about other contraceptive provision.

- Record a log of IUD and IUS fittings and their outcomes.
- Record in your reflective diary changes you have made to your provision of contraception.
- Re-audit the availability and adequacy of emergency resuscitation equipment after any necessary changes have been made, and also record the training standards of health professionals who use it.
- Record that you set aside a longer appointment time for patients (with their consent) because you were teaching e.g. demonstrating counselling and insertion techniques for an IUD or implant fitting as in the case study.
- Record how you helped the registrar learn from managing Mrs Daffy himself, rather than just taking over completely yourself.

Box 5.7:   Case study continued

It is clearly impossible to undertake an adequate medical assessment initially. Help the GP registrar to arrange with Mrs Daffy for someone to look after the children while he does this assessment. If it is beyond the limits of the GP registrar's competence, he may need to refer Mrs Daffy to another health professional for contraceptive treatment.

Mrs Daffy refused the offer of an immediate injection or pill. She was able to get her sister to look after the older children, while she just brought the baby to the surgery. One of the receptionists was able to look after the baby after he had been fed and was in his pushchair. The registrar was able to have a full discussion of the options for contraception. She said her husband would never 'be done'. She decided she definitely wanted an IUS after all the advantages and disadvantages were explained. She was keen for the registrar to see the IUS fitting which the registrar's trainer was able to do the following week.

The GP registrar will probably want to discuss Mrs Daffy's situation with the health visitor and should ask her for permission to do so. Other professionals, such as a social worker, might be involved with the family.

References

1   Department of Health (1999) *Teenage Pregnancy.* Social Exclusion Unit, Department of Health, London.

2   Chambers R, Wakley G and Chambers S (2001) *Tackling Teenage Pregnancy: sex culture and needs.* Radcliffe Medical Press, Oxford.

3   Acheson D (chair) (1998) *Independent Inquiry into Inequalities in Health Report.* The Stationery Office, London.

4   The general leaflet *Contraception*, those on individual methods, and a good range of other leaflets, are available from fpa, 2–12 Pentonville Road, London N1 9FP, UK; telephone: +44 (0)20 7837 5432.

5   http://www.who.int/reproductive-health and World Health Organization (2000) *Improving Access to Quality Care in Family Planning.* WHO, Geneva.

6   http://www.ffprhc.org.uk/.

7   Faculty of Family Planning and Reproductive Health Care: Clinical Effectiveness Unit (2003) FFPRHC guidance: emergency contraception. *J Fam Plann & RHC.* **29(2)**: 9–16.

8   Trussel J (1998) Contraceptive efficacy. In: J Trussel, F Stewart, W Cates, GK Stewart, D Kowal and F Guest F (eds). *Contraceptive Technology* (17e). Ardent Media, New York.

9   Belfield T (1999) *Contraceptive Handbook* (3e). Family Planning Association, London.

10 Ellertson C, Evans M, Ferden S *et al.* (2003) Extending the time limit for starting the Yupze regimen of emergency contraception to 120 hours. *Obstet Gynecol.* **101(6)**: 1168–71.

11 von Hertzen H, Piaggio G, Ding J *et al.* (2002) Low dose mifepristone and two regimens of levonorgestrel for emergency contraception: a WHO multicentre randomised trial. *Lancet.* **360(9348)**: 1803–10.

Further reading

- Belfield T (1999) *Contraceptive Handbook* (3e). Family Planning Association, London.
- Guillebaud J (1999) *Contraception: your questions answered.* Churchill Livingstone, London.
- Rowlands S (1997) *Managing Family Planning in General Practice.* Radcliffe Medical Press, Oxford.
- Royal College of Obstetricians and Gynaecologists (1998) *Male and Female Sterilisation.* Royal College of Obstetricians and Gynaecologists, London.
- Wakley G and Chambers R (2002) *Sexual Health Matters in Primary Care.* Radcliffe Medical Press, Oxford.
- Wakley G, Cunnion M and Chambers R (2003) *Improving Sexual Health Advice.* Radcliffe Medical Press, Oxford.

6

Sexually transmitted infections

Box 6.1: Case study

A 21-year-old woman attends your surgery telling you that her recent ex-partner has sent her a text message accusing her of giving him an infection. She has little other information except that he has been to the genitourinary medicine (GUM) clinic in the next town. She refuses to attend the GUM clinic and wants you to treat her.

What issues you should cover[1]

Giving information about genitourinary (GUM) clinics

Access to GUM clinics varies across the country and new users often find it difficult to know what is available. People are often fearful of attending because of perceived stigma, or just because going somewhere new always provokes anxiety – and it is difficult to ask a friend to go with them for support. You should know where the clinics are and how people can be seen. Some clinics have open access while others require appointments to be made by telephone. Some are open in the evening, others from 10am to 5pm (not very convenient!). Some of the clinics now have a seamless one-stop service together with contraceptive clinics or are on the same premises to allow for easy transfers between services.

Stress that the service is confidential and that the records are kept separately from other hospital records. By law, staff in a GUM clinic cannot tell a patient if or what sexually transmitted infection (STI) their partner has, or tell their doctor that they have attended unless the patient requests it. The clinic cannot give any information to other doctors, solicitors, insurance companies or the police without the consent of the patient. The clinic will record a name and a date of birth, and will ask for a contact address so that results can be given (but patients do not have to give this information if they prefer not to).

After a detailed history, often using a checklist, tests can be done immediately to diagnose some infections. Other tests will take some time for the results to be known. The clinic does need some identifying information so that they can access patients' records when they re-attend. All treatment is free of charge and this can be a potent incentive to attend if treatment is needed. Reimbursement of travel expenses can also sometimes be made.

The patient needs to be clear that you will not be able to give such a complete service in general practice, partly because of your limitations for carrying out testing. Results of testing are more reliable if the patient travels to the hospital laboratory with her samples still in her in the body than if you take samples and transport them separately. The pick up rate from samples falls the longer the delay between testing and examination of the specimens.

Taking a sexual history[1]

If she still refuses to attend the GUM clinic, then you must do your best for her. Explain the reason for taking a sexual history. This reduces the possibility that the patient will be offended or misinterpret your intentions. Ask the patient if it is all right to carry on.

Tell the patient about confidentiality – mention this early on and explain how the information given will be kept confidential and who will have access to that information. Consider asking their partner to participate or to supply information if the patient agrees (unlikely in this case). If a partner does attend, allow for one-to-one discussion, as some issues involve sexual activity with other partners or information that one of a couple would not want the other to hear.

Listen carefully – allow the patient to guide the discussion and introduce the terminology. This does not imply that you should use the same language or slang as patients do. Be careful about the words that you and the patient use. The vagina or uterus mean something specific to you, but the terms may be used in a much wider sense by patients to indicate any part of the female genitals. Similarly, someone may talk about 'going to bed with someone' and you need to be clear whether this actually includes sexual penetration. 'Making love' may include sexual penetration, or may refer to caressing and other sexual stimulation. There are problems too with identifying the sex of the partner; 'Pat' or 'Lesley' could be either. Always check that what you understand is what the patient meant.

Ask the patient to tell you about her sexual activity. Give examples e.g. have you had oral sex? Explain each time why you are asking those questions. Other forms of sexual activity should also be specified, depending on the patient's sexual orientation. You will need to know the areas of the body that might become infected (throat, rectum, etc.) so that investigations are complete but relevant.

Ask about symptoms, but bear in mind (and tell the patient) that most people with an STI do not have any symptoms. Has she had any burning when she passes water, any change in her vaginal secretions, any soreness, rash or lumps in the genital area or any irregular bleeding between the periods or after intercourse? Has there been any change in the amount of her period loss or any episodes of abdominal pain?

Enquire about any previous STI and her own perception of her risk. An estimate can be made from the length of time she was with that partner and how many other sexual partners she has had in the last 12 months.

Give information about STIs

You need to find out what she knows about STIs. She may be reluctant to have any investigations performed if she has no symptoms. You can give her some information about how often people are infected in her age group and about her risks – adjusted for her level of comprehension. Then she will be in a better position to make an informed choice.

Statistics about STIs[2]

Cases of chlamydia trachomatis identified have doubled in the last six years. In 2000, genital chlamydial infection was the commonest bacterial STI seen. Highest rates of diagnosis of chlamydia are seen in young people, particularly women in the 16–19 year and 20–24 year age groups.

Genital warts (HPV) are the commonest viral STI and also the commonest STI overall.

Gonorrhoea (GC): the rise in the number of cases of gonorrhoea has been largest in the youngest age groups – 16–19 years and 20–24 years of age. The majority of cases identified have been in men – largely because women rarely have symptoms.

Genital herpes first attack rates have risen slightly. The rise in the numbers of new cases of syphilis that recently occurred was mainly in men who have sex with men.

Human immunodeficiency virus (HIV) infection rates continue to rise. HIV infection is now identified more commonly in heterosexuals than in homosexual men. Infection rates are increasing, perhaps due to a relaxation of the vigilance of people who believed that they were at risk and used condoms after publicity campaigns, but have now become complacent about the risk, as it is no longer in the news.

Hepatitis B (HBV) rates have slightly decreased but hepatitis C (HCV) rates have increased, perhaps reflecting the effect of immunisation against hepatitis B.

Some other infections that occur elsewhere in the body such as strepto-coccus (which usually causes skin and throat infections), or gut bacteria like *E. coli*, can be spread by sexual activity. Molluscum contagiosum is a very common infection, especially in children but can also be spread through sexual activity. Some other more unusual STIs may be seen occasionally in people returning from other countries.

Although thrush and bacterial vaginosis are not classified as STIs, they are common causes of genital infection. Thrush (also known as candida, or candidiasis) is not usually passed on from a woman to a man by sexual inter-course. It is a very common cause of vaginal discharge, soreness and itching. Bacterial vaginosis is possibly even more frequently found in women com-plaining of vaginal discharge.

Knowledge about the individual infections[3]

Ask her what she knows about the infections to find out what other informa-tion she might need.

Chlamydia

In under-26 year olds, chlamydia has been identified in about 10–12% of people in pilot studies of population screening. Chlamydial infection is frequently asymptomatic but is a common cause of infertility and chronic pelvic infection. It can cause ectopic pregnancy and chronic pelvic pain. Ascending infection in men causes epididymitis but evidence of male infertility is limited. Maternal to infant transmission causes neonatal conjunctivitis and pneumonia. It may co-exist with other STIs and may help in the transmission and acquisition of HIV infection.

Gonorrhoea

The incidence of this infection is increasing especially among 16–19 year olds. Infection can be asymptomatic in about 10% of men and 50% of women. Male symptoms of dysuria, discharge or epididymitis, or female symptoms of discharge, dysuria or abdominal pain should raise your suspicions.

Non-specific urethritis or non-specific genital infection

This is common in young men and is defined as an infection, usually urethritis, not caused by gonorrhoea. Up to 40% of episodes of urethritis are in fact caused by chlamydia, so she will need tests for this. *Mycoplasma genitalium* and *Ureaplasma urealyticum* are commonest among the other causative organisms. The diagnosis is mainly made by a combination of symptoms of urethritis and the presence of pus cells – more than five per high power field (×400) – on a slide made from a urethral swab. The male partner will have been told to get his partner(s) treated to prevent recurrence. Treatment is as for chlamydia.

Genital warts – human papilloma virus (HPV)

First ever presentation of genital warts has shown a significant rise in the 16–19 year old age group. HPV infection is common among sexually active young people whether or not visible warts are present. Small plane warts may be visible on examination without any symptoms being present. Genital warts are usually spread sexually, so their presence should prompt a search for other STIs. Some HPVs (types 16, 18, 31, 33 and 35) – not usually the ones presenting as visible warts – are associated with the development of cervical cancer and yearly cervical screening for five years is normally suggested if wart virus is found. Determining the type of HPV present is still a research technique.

Syphilis

Although many people know that syphilis is an STI, new cases of syphilis in the UK are uncommon and are mostly found by screening in pregnancy or on blood donation. The presence of a solitary ulcer or the rash of secondary syphilis may raise suspicions.

Viral hepatitis

Several different virus types cause hepatitis, all of which can cause an acute illness with jaundice. Asymptomatic infections are common. Hepatitis B, C and D also cause chronic infection progressing to cirrhosis and liver failure. Hepatitis B is more infectious than HIV and can be spread by sexual intercourse as well as from contaminated blood. Hepatitis A can be caught sexually from a partner with an active infection.

Human immunodeficiency disease (HIV)

The symptoms of an acute infection with HIV may resemble glandular fever, but most new infections do not show any symptoms. The development of antibodies after infection takes about two to six weeks, but can be later than this. Chronic infection may also be asymptomatic, but about one-third of patients have generalised persistently enlarged lymph nodes. Later in the course of the chronic infection, symptoms of night sweats, fevers, diarrhoea and weight loss occur. Frequent infections of mucous membranes or skin are often present.

About 75% of HIV-positive people develop symptoms over a 9–10 year period without therapy.

Trichomonas vaginalis

This organism with a flagella occurs in the urethra in both genders but also in the vagina and paraurethral glands in women. In adults it is a sexually transmitted infection and is frequently associated with other STIs (babies can acquire the infection perinatally from an infected mother). The commonest complaint in both men and women is of discharge, but 15–50% of infected men have no symptoms. Women also complain of itching, dysuria or a smelly discharge. Although the discharge is classically described as frothy yellow, it is often variable both in consistency and colour.

Bacterial vaginosis

Bacterial vaginosis (BV) may be even more common than 'thrush'. It was formerly called 'Gardnerella vaginosis' and is the overgrowth of predominately anaerobic bacteria that are normally present in only small numbers in the healthy vagina. They produce a fishy or ammonia smell in alkaline conditions so the condition may be worse after intercourse or just after a woman's periods have finished.

BV is causing increasing concern to health professionals because of:

- pelvic inflammatory disease
- endometritis
- postoperative cuff infection after a transabdominal hysterectomy (TAH) and vaginal hysterectomy
- postabortal infection
- psychosexual problems (the smell!)
- obstetric factors:
  - increase in late miscarriage rates
  - chorioendometritis
  - pre-term delivery
- being a possible co-factor in HIV transmission.

Thrush

Sometimes this fungal infection may be reported on cervical smears or swabs taken for other reasons when there are no symptoms. The first attack can be extremely uncomfortable with the swelling, itching, soreness and discharge causing considerable distress. Although often described as typically presenting with white 'cottage cheese' like patches over bright red areas of the vulval or vaginal walls, this is more frequent in pregnancy. The appearance of the discharge may be very variable and the vulva may be fissured or red and shiny from frequent scratching. Most women complain mainly of:

- itching and soreness
- rapid onset often in the pre-menstrual week
- painful urination and/or sexual intercourse.

Investigations that may be needed

You need to discuss with the woman what tests you can do, how long the results will take and how she will obtain the results. She may be happy for you to contact her at home but, if not, other arrangements must be made such as sending them to a trusted friend. If she does not give consent to be contacted then it is essential that she understands that she must re-attend for the results.

Table 6.1:   Suggested investigations for screening for an STI indicated by the history

Test	Useful for
High vaginal swab (HVS) in Stuart's or similar transport medium	Candida, bacterial vaginosis, trichomonas
Cervical exudate swab or endocervical swab and urethral swab in Stuart's or similar transport medium	Gram stain shows gram-negative diplococcus in about half of all gonococcal infections; culture as well will detect about 90% of infections
Chlamydia test Know which testing procedure your microbiology department uses. If it is enzyme immunoassay (EIA) send an endocervical swab and urethral swab. Use the special chlamydial testing kit supplied by your laboratory for taking samples from the cervix. Follow the instructions that come with the pack from the laboratory as each type of pack has different instructions. Some are very clear and state that the cleaning swab (the large bulbous swab of the two) must not be used as the swab for chlamydia. First clean any mucus off the cervix with the cleaning swab and then use the chlamydia swab (the metal- or plastic-handled, thin flat-ended swab). Rotate it for a minimum of 30 seconds in the cervix. Take cells from the transitional zone (the junction between the outer cells of the cervix and the inner ones lining the cervical canal). Remove the swab from the vagina and place it in the container supplied in accordance with the instructions.	Chlamydia trachomatis

continued overleaf

Table 6.1: *continued*

Test	Useful for
First catch urine (*not* midstream (MSU))	Nucleic acid amplification tests for chlamydia trachomatis*
Viral swabs from any ulcers or sores	Herpes simplex, candida
Swabs from other sites e.g. pharynx, rectum	Gonococcus
Blood test	Viral hepatitis or HIV

Nucleic acid amplification tests have been developed that are highly sensitive (over 90%) compared with the standard endocervical EIA test that has a lower sensitivity of 60–70%. You will need to know what the standards are for your laboratory and their specificity rate (so that you know how many false-positive and false-negative results might be expected).

Prevention of transmission[4]

It is important to ensure that any infection is not spread to any other partner(s). Partner notification is an important part of the control of STIs but is often difficult to achieve. The woman should be advised to abstain from intercourse until she has been screened and treated. Remember that not all women are able to refuse to have sexual intercourse if there is an imbalance of power between the partners, or if cultural or religious customs prevent her expressing her wishes.

Treatment[5]

If you can establish what infection her previous partner has been told he has, treatment for this infection could be started as soon as investigations are complete. She should only be treated empirically if you cannot obtain her consent to investigations. It is possible for her to have an infection that has not been identified in her previous partner. The reasons for this can be either that he has not contracted an infection that she has, or because of the limitations of the test (that is, he has had a false-negative test).

General principles to consider when introducing screening of well people for illnesses or infections

---

Box 6.2:   Case study continued

Before she leaves, the patient asks you why she was not screened for infections like chlamydia when she had her recent cervical smear. You tell her a little of what is described in Box 6.3 and the general principles of screening with special regard to chlamydia.

Box 6.3:   General principles to consider when screening for illnesses or infections

- Is the condition important?
  – chlamydia is an important cause of infertility, ectopic pregnancy, salpingitis, chronic pelvic pain and morbidity

- Is the natural history well understood?
  – 70–80% of women have cervical infections with no symptoms, but it is not clear how many have a risk of ascending infections in the absence of precipitating factors such as instrumentation of the uterus

- Is there a recognisable early stage?
  – screening tests can identify infection when no symptoms are present

- Is there a suitable test?
  – the nucleic acid amplification tests are more sensitive and specific than the previous enzyme immunoassay tests and can be done on urine as well as swabs. Blood tests are not useful as they tell you only if someone has ever had the infection (and possibly got rid of it) not whether they have it currently

- Is the test acceptable?
  – urine tests are more acceptable than cervical or urethral swabs. Self-taken swabs have also been shown to be useful and acceptable in some groups

- At what intervals should the test be repeated?
  – unknown – and may depend on the accuracy and completeness of contact tracing and treatment, and on social factors like change of sexual partner or monogamy

- Are there adequate facilities for the diagnosis and treatment?
  – no: primary care health professionals do not always have sufficient time or skills or facilities for investigation, GUM clinics need increased resources to cope with the number of referrals of people with positive

continued overleaf

tests, the laboratories have insufficient capacity and resources to carry out the tests. Instigating a campaign about chlamydia screening without increasing the facilities for screening, further testing for confirmation and for treatment would cause collapse of the present already overstretched arrangements

- Is treatment at an early stage of more benefit than treatment at a later stage?

  – definitely – infection can easily be eradicated in the early stages before structural damage occurs. However, it is unknown how often people recover from chlamydial infection without treatment[6]

- Are the chances of physical and psychological harm less than the chances of benefit?

  – this depends on how the test is presented, people's feelings about stigmatisation (having a 'sexually transmitted infection') and public knowledge about the condition

- Can the cost be balanced against the benefits the service provides, versus other opportunity costs and benefits?

  – unknown as yet: early pilot studies from Merseyside[7] and Southampton[8] showed much higher prevalence of infection and higher costs for the counselling time and number of tests performed than expected. Further pilots at ten sites are ongoing.

You can read about setting up your own guidelines that might be part of a development plan in your workplace in the book *Sexual Health Matters in Primary Care*.[1]

Managing infection control in general practice

You clear up your swabbing equipment after the patient has left and consider whether you have removed all trace of infection. If you're unsure you could consider using the interactive CD ROM based on the BMA's published guidelines (1998) on blood borne viruses (HIV, HBV, HCV) that is available from the BMA.[9] Key issues covered include: infection prevention, decontamination methods, safe handling and disposal of sharps, and post-exposure prophylaxis. The Department of Health, Medical Devices Agency and Health and Safety Executive assisted in the development of the material.[10] Your practice team could audit knowledge and procedures before and after its use.

Collecting data to demonstrate your learning, competence, performance and standards of service delivery: sexually transmitted infections

Example cycle of evidence 6.1

- Focus: clinical care
- Other relevant focus of evidence: relationships with patients

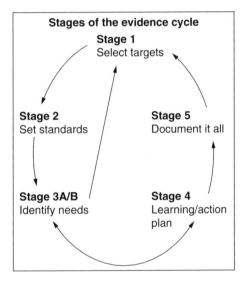

Stages of the evidence cycle

Stage 1
Select targets

Stage 2
Set standards

Stage 5
Document it all

Stage 3A/B
Identify needs

Stage 4
Learning/action plan

Box 6.4:   Case study

Miss Fret attends with 'lumps down below'. You insist that you are chaperoned by the practice nurse while you examine her, although she says it doesn't bother her. She has several vulval warts and you refer her with a letter to the GUM clinic for screening (in case she has other STIs) and treatment. She contacts you, distressed even more, as she cannot get an appointment at the GUM clinic for three weeks.

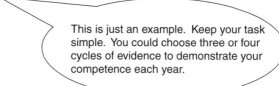

This is just an example. Keep your task simple. You could choose three or four cycles of evidence to demonstrate your competence each year.

Stage 1: Select your aspirations for good practice

The excellent GP:

- provides or arranges investigations or treatment when necessary
- takes suitable and prompt action when required
- refers to another practitioner when indicated
- does not allow beliefs to influence the advice or treatment provided, or if beliefs are likely to affect patient management tells patients of their right to see another doctor
- makes efficient use of resources, but records, reports and endeavours to rectify deficiencies in resources
- empowers patients to take decisions about their management.

Stage 2: Set the standards for your outcomes

Outcomes might include:

- the way learning is applied
- a learnt skill
- a protocol
- a strategy that is implemented
- meeting recommended standards.

- Demonstrate consistent best practice in provision of investigation and treatment of suspected STIs in respect of availability and accessibility and clinical management.

Stage 3A: Identify your learning needs

- Carry out a self-assessment of your knowledge about the investigation of STIs.
- Conduct a significant event audit e.g. a young woman who developed pelvic inflammatory disease three months after she failed to attend the GUM clinic after you gave her a referral letter.

- Keep a reflective diary capturing trends or comments relating to problems dealing with the sexual activity of young women.
- Reflect on your previous insistence that Miss Fret is examined in the presence of the practice nurse and whether you were imposing your views (and fears) on her.

Stage 3B: Identify your service needs

> Any of the needs assessment exercises in 3A may also reveal service needs.

- Record the pathway of care when young women consult you or other health professionals with sexually related complaints.
- Collect data about access and arrangements for referral to the GUM clinic.

Stage 4: Make and carry out a learning and action plan

- Compare your knowledge of the investigation and management of STIs in young women with an authoritative source you obtain and read.
- Prepare a draft practice guideline for the investigation and management of STIs.
- Obtain statistics about the workload and waiting times at the nearest GUM clinic and how you can make representations to try to improve the availability of services.

Stage 5: Document your learning, competence, performance and standards of service delivery

- Collect feedback from the GUM clinic about service delivery.
- Collect feedback from other health professionals about your draft guidelines for the investigation and management of STIs.
- Keep extracts of information from your reflective diary about your greater understanding of young women's sexual behaviour and the changes you have made so that you feel that your attitude is not perceived as judgemental or defensive.

Box 6.5:   Case study continued

Miss Fret is naturally anxious and unhappy about the management of her problems. You need to discuss with her how the situation can be managed. You are able to offer Miss Fret a morning consultation for collecting samples for investigation. She takes them to the hospital herself to ensure their rapid transport. No other STI is found. The practice nurse is willing to repeatedly paint the warts with podophyllin, which Miss Fret washes off after three hours. The practice nurse passes on Miss Fret's thanks (and you record this in your portfolio!).

Example cycle of evidence 6.2

- Focus: maintaining good medical practice
- Other relevant focus of evidence: working with colleagues

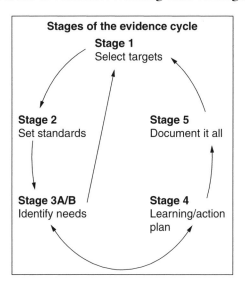

Stages of the evidence cycle

Stage 1
Select targets

Stage 2
Set standards

Stage 5
Document it all

Stage 3A/B
Identify needs

Stage 4
Learning/action plan

Box 6.6:   Case study

Mrs Rabbit had been screened for STIs following a diagnosis of non-specific urethritis (NSU) in her current partner. You do not have access to urine testing in your area and EIA testing from a cervical swab did not pick up any infection. You explain to her that as a contact she should be treated and decide on a prescription for a seven day course of oxytetracyline. Just as you are printing out the prescription, you notice that she saw one of the other doctors in the practice yesterday. You feel annoyed that this other doctor did not deal with this problem, as the results were available then. Then you notice that a pregnancy test has been sent off.

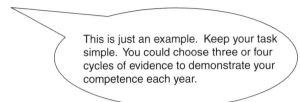

This is just an example. Keep your task simple. You could choose three or four cycles of evidence to demonstrate your competence each year.

Stage 1: Select your aspirations for good practice

The excellent GP:

- works with colleagues to monitor and maintain the quality of care provided
- is continually aware of patient safety
- takes part in regular and systematic clinical audits and makes improvements accordingly
- takes part in confidential enquiries, adverse event recognition and reporting, to help reduce risks to patients
- does not allow personal opinions about colleagues' personal characteristics to affect professional relationships
- respects the skills and contributions of colleagues.

Stage 2: Set the standards for your outcomes

Outcomes might include:

- the way learning is applied
- a learnt skill
- a protocol
- a strategy that is implemented
- meeting recommended standards.

- Demonstrate consistent best practice for the management of test results within the practice.
- Demonstrate consistent best practice in the prevention of harm to patients from potential prescribing errors.

Stage 3A: Identify your learning needs

- Reflect on how best to approach colleagues with whom you feel irritated about clinical matters or non-clinical issues.
- Review your knowledge of the sensitivity and specificity of the tests (in this case in relation to sexual health) being used by your laboratory so that you understand fully the likelihood of a patient having a false-positive or false-negative result.

- Reflect on whether your own personality makes it difficult for colleagues to act on your behalf. Are you too possessive of 'your' patients, wanting to undertake all their care? Can you demonstrate shared care for other patients who have been seen by other health professionals?
- Ask for some anonymous feedback on your teamworking skills. Do you feel that your experience or knowledge makes you a 'better' doctor (or just one with different skills and knowledge)?

Stage 3B: Identify your service needs

> Any of the needs assessment exercises in 3A may also reveal service needs.

- Undertake a significant event audit where a prescribing error was made, with the rest of the clinicians in the practice team.
- Find out how results of investigations are currently managed.
- Reflect on how you all inform other members of the team about what you have done, and how you find out what is happening. Do you need to increase your communication skills or use of internal email or make more effort to attend practice meetings?

Stage 4: Make and carry out a learning and action plan

- Find out how other practices manage the results of investigations before making proposals at the practice meeting.
- Find out how to add an alert to the prescribing module and add one about checking for pregnancy before prescribing.
- Revisit the guidelines on treatment of NSU and chlamydia in women who are, or are not, pregnant.[6]
- Research the data about completion of treatment courses and decide whether an alternative treatment (such as azithromycin as a single dose) would be more cost-effective than oxytetracyline as a four times a day course for seven days.

Stage 5: Document your learning, competence, performance and standards of service delivery

- Record how results will be managed by the practice and plan an audit to look at how the changes are working.
- Record how the alert was added to the prescribing module.
- Show how you disseminated your learning about cost-effective treatments to others.

Box 6.7:   Case study continued

You are made aware of possible conflicts in the management of this patient. You just avoided prescribing oxytetracyline for a patient who is possibly pregnant. You were able to prevent an adverse event by your prompt action in changing Mrs Rabbit's medication. You added an alert that reminded you to check for the risk of pregnancy whenever prescribing tetracylines to women. You tactfully discussed the difficulties of dealing with other people's investigation results in a practice meeting and obtained a consensus decision for better management in the future.

Example cycle of evidence 6.3

- Focus: research
- Other relevant focus of evidence: management

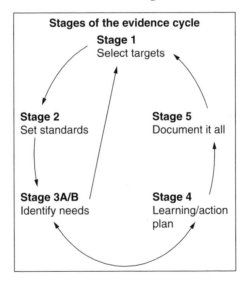

Stages of the evidence cycle

Stage 1
Select targets

Stage 2
Set standards

Stage 5
Document it all

Stage 3A/B
Identify needs

Stage 4
Learning/action plan

Box 6.8:   Case study

Dr Leap and Dr Jump want to apply for funding to introduce screening for chlamydia and to be able to offer routine testing for HIV in their practice. They want to be able to show that the service they provide is enhanced by these measures and that the uptake of both services justifies the investment. Their intention is to use a questionnaire to find out the level of knowledge that their service users and staff have, then provide education, information and training as appropriate, so that they can introduce the new services. They will measure the level of knowledge again and the uptake of the new services.

This is just an example. Keep your task simple. You could choose three or four cycles of evidence to demonstrate your competence each year.

Stage 1: Select your aspirations for good practice

The excellent GP:

- puts the care and safety of patients first when participating in research
- conducts all research in an ethical manner, with honesty and integrity
- is satisfied that the foreseeable risks will not outweigh the potential benefits to patients, in therapeutic research
- is satisfied that the potential benefits from the development of treatments and furthering of knowledge far outweigh any foreseeable risks to participants, in non-therapeutic research
- completes, if possible, research projects involving patients or volunteers or ensures that they are completed by others (except where harms or risks are expected)
- ensures that care is provided and supervised by staff who have appropriate levels of competence
- ensures that working methods and the working environment conform to health and safety legislation and that safe working practices are followed
- monitors and reviews the quality of the care provided in the work environment.

Stage 2: Set the standards for your outcomes

Outcomes might include:

- the way learning is applied
- a learnt skill
- a protocol
- a strategy that is implemented
- meeting recommended standards.

- Demonstrate consistent best practice in carrying out the research project.
- Demonstrate consistent best practice in the provision of information, teaching and training, and service provision regarding the research project.

- Monitor staff's successful completion of a specific education and training programme.
- All blood products should be assumed to be potentially injurious and handled accordingly. A protocol for needle-stick injuries is in place.[9]

Stage 3A: Identify your learning needs

- Find or select a suitable questionnaire to use in an audit of health professionals' knowledge and attitudes about HIV.
- Establish how to write the protocol for the research project and obtain ethical approval. Plan how you will analyse, collate and write up the findings.

Stage 3B: Identify your service needs

Any of the needs assessment exercises in 3A may also reveal service needs.

- Establish the needs of both staff and patients for information, and of the staff for education and training.
- Manage the changeover from investigating chlamydia to screening for it (*see* Box 6.3).
- Determine how to manage the change to offering HIV testing to all as a routine and the confidentiality issues involved.

Stage 4: Make and carry out a learning and action plan

- Refresh research skills and bring them up to date.
- Understand the current requirements for ethical approval.
- Learn more about change management at a workshop.
- Work together to examine the literature and draw up the protocol.
- Read a book or articles about completing research studies.
- Visit other clinics or surgeries already providing these services.

Stage 5: Document your learning, competence, performance and standards of service delivery

- Record the progress with the project as the stages are worked through.
- Write up the project together when complete.
- Re-audit the level of knowledge among staff and patients.
- Keep a copy of research ethics approval and permission from the PCO to host the research.
- Keep a copy of the evaluation of the project.

Box 6.9: Case study continued

Dr Leap and Dr Jump quickly abandon the idea of introducing screening for chlamydia because they discover that they would have to wait for funding until the reports from the pilot schemes for screening were available. They establish low levels of knowledge among both patients and staff about HIV testing, and after an enthusiastic campaign of information and staff training are able to introduce routine testing for HIV. Their figures show a low level of uptake during the first six months, but a much better uptake by the second six months.

References

1 Wakley G and Chambers R (2002) *Sexual Health Matters in Primary Care.* Radcliffe Medical Press, Oxford

2 The most recently available statistics on STIs are available from http://www.hpa.org.uk/infections/default.htm.

3 Adler MW (1999) *ABC of Sexually Transmitted Diseases.* BMJ Publishing Group, London.

4 Godlee F (ed.) (2003) *Clinical Evidence.* BMJ Publishing Group, London. http://www.clinicalevidence.com.

5 Joint Formulary Committee (2003) *British National Formulary.* British Medical Association and Royal Pharmaceutical Society of Great Britain, London. Also at http://www.bnf.org.

6 Godlee F (ed.) (2003) Genital chlamydial infection. *Clin Evid.* **9**: 1721–7.

7 Harvey J, Webb A and Mallinson H (2000) *Chlamydia trachomatis* screening in young people in Merseyside. *Br J Fam Plann.* **26(4)**: 199–201.

8 Basarab A, Browning D, Lanham S and O'Connell S (2002) Pilot study to assess the presence of *Chlamydia trachomatis* in urine from 18–30-year-old males using EIA/IF and PCR. *J Fam Plann & RHC.* **28(1)**: 36–7.

9 Board of Science and Education, British Medical Association (1998) *Bloodborne Viruses and Infection Control: a guide for health care professionals.* Interactive CD ROM. BMJ Books, London.

10 Department of Health (2000) *HIV Post-Exposure Prophylaxis: Guidance from the UK Chief Medical Officers' Expert Advisory Group on AIDS.* Department of Health, London.

Further reading and other sources of information

- Avert (UK based charity giving extensive AIDS information) www.avert.org.
- Carter Y, Moss C and Weyman A (eds) (1998) *RCGP Handbook of Sexual Health in Primary Care.* Royal College of General Practitioners, London.
- Chief Medical Officer's expert advisory group report on chlamydia www.doh.gov.uk/chlamyd.htm.
- Department of Health National Strategy for Sexual Health and HIV www.doh.gov.uk/nshs/index.htm.
- Genitourinary infections and GUM clinic list www.agum.org.uk.
- *Guidelines* – summarising clinical guidelines for primary care (latest issue). Representatives of professional bodies and organisations producing guidelines. Medendium Group Publishing Ltd, Berkhamstead. Also at http://www.eguidelines.co.uk. This gives you the source for the full guidelines for any particular condition.
- Members of the BMA Foundation for AIDS (2002) *Take the HIV Test.* Medical Foundation for AIDS and Sexual Health, BMA House, Tavistock Square, London WC1H 9JP. Website: http://www.medfash.org.uk.
- Scottish Intercollegiate Guidelines Network (SIGN) www.sign.ac.uk.
- *STI Online* includes issues of *Sexually Transmitted Infections* published since 1967 and includes *Genitourinary Medicine* and the *British Journal of Venereal Diseases.* http://sti.bmjjournals.com.
- Wakley G, Cunnion M and Chambers R (2003) *Improving Sexual Health Advice.* Radcliffe Medical Press, Oxford.

7

Infertility in general practice

An infertility consultation may take some time to cover all the relevant issues. Thus it may be wise at the start of the consultation to agree what you will cover and perhaps arrange a further consultation with more time. At the initial consultation the first priority is to provide some prognostic information reassuring the couple that although infertility is common, most couples will ultimately achieve a pregnancy. Secondly, it is important to take this opportunity for pre-pregnancy assessment to optimise the outlook for a healthy pregnancy and normal baby. Specific assessment regarding infertility should be commenced in a systematic fashion. An enthusiastic GP can go a long way to establishing a diagnosis and steering a couple's management appropriately.[1]

Box 7.1: Case study

Mrs Brie, a 32-year-old woman who has recently registered with your practice, attends with her 43-year-old husband seeking advice, as they are concerned that they have not achieved a pregnancy after trying for six months. Mrs Brie is a hairdresser with a passion for soft cheeses and her husband is a sheep farmer, who has been pleased with the expansion of his farm in the last few years. They had a miscarriage three years earlier which they found very distressing and it has taken them some time to decide to try for a further pregnancy.

Mrs Brie has read on the Internet that dietary changes can have a major impact on fertility. You suspect Mrs Brie's passion for food may extend beyond soft cheese as she weighs 80 kg at a height of 1.6 m (BMI 31). Her menstrual cycle is regular at 28 days duration and she notices midcycle abdominal discomfort when her cervical mucus also seems more profuse.

What issues you should cover

Even before arranging any tests, it is possible to give the couple useful prognostic information by considering their age, duration of infertility and any prior pregnancies.[2] Although it may be tempting to reassure the couple that six months is too soon to worry, it is important first to establish how long the couple have been having intercourse without contraception. Couples may stop contraception without actively trying for a pregnancy and only regard the period of infertility as the time that they were actively trying for pregnancy. Although fertility declines with female age, at 32 years the outlook remains good. The influence of male age is much less marked. As the couple have achieved a pregnancy in the past, they are likely to achieve a further pregnancy, even though the previous pregnancy did not lead to a baby.

The couple may find it useful for you to give them some idea of the average time to conception based on their circumstances. It is possible to calculate this from Tables 7.1 and 7.2 or using the fertility calculator on the Internet.[3]

Such calculators only provide a guide and individual circumstances may alter the prognosis. In this case, Mrs Brie is obese which may have an adverse influence even though she appears to be ovulating. She certainly should be encouraged to lose weight, setting realistic targets for weight loss.

Mrs Brie has particular risks from toxoplasmosis from the sheep and listeria from soft cheeses. It is important to explain this without causing undue alarm and suggest simple measures such as avoidance of soft cheeses, and the sheep, particularly at lambing time.

Table 7.1:   A guide to prognosis for pregnancy without fertility treatment: average baseline prognosis[2]

Months	Cumulative live birth rate (%)
3	4.2
6	8.1
12	14.3
24	21.2
36	25.2

Table 7.2:   A guide to prognosis for pregnancy without fertility treatment: effects of prognostic factors[2]

Prognostic factor	Multiplication factor
Prior pregnancy in partnership	1.8
Duration of infertility <36 months	1.7
Female age <30 years	1.5
Male defect	0.5
Endometriosis	0.4
Tubal defect	0.5

The baseline cumulative pregnancy rate is modified by applying each multiplication factor that applies to the couple, providing an individualised chance of pregnancy. For instance if a couple had one prior pregnancy, multiplying the baseline rate by 1.8 would increase their cumulative live birth rate. If a couple had a prior pregnancy and had endometriosis, then the baseline rate would be multiplied by 1.8 times 0.4.

A general approach to the initial assessment of the infertile couple is outlined in the guidelines of the Royal College of Obstetricians and Gynaecologists (RCOG) (*see* Figure 7.1).

Unexplained infertility

In many cases, initial assessment may uncover no specific cause for infertility. Even after comprehensive assessment, around one in four couples' infertility may be classified as 'unexplained'.[5]

Box 7.2:   Case study continued

Mr and Mrs Brie return to your surgery with the results of their initial investigations. Although initially following the miscarriage the couple had used condoms, they had stopped using any contraception over 14 months previously. Mrs Brie has joined a local dieting club and since you last saw her six weeks previously she has lost 3 kg in weight. She has found this very difficult to achieve and wonders if there is any treatment she could have to help her to lose further weight.

It is important to provide the couple with reassurance and support explaining the likelihood of conception if they persevere. As the couple have over one year's infertility it is reasonable to refer to them to the local fertility clinic, particularly if the waiting list is long, as this secures their place in the 'queue' to be seen.

Weight reduction will not only benefit the chance of achieving a pregnancy but will also improve the outlook for any pregnancy and have wider health benefits. The National electronic Library for Health provides guidance on weight reduction, including the place for medications (or look back to Chapter 4).[6]

Mixed tubal and male factor infertility

In many cases there are multiple infertility factors often affecting both the male and female side. It is thus always important to manage a couple together

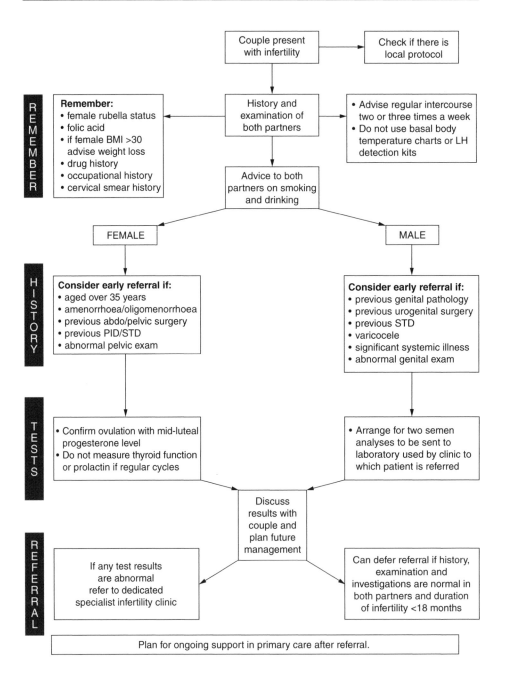

Figure 7.1: Recommendations for initial assessment of the infertile couple (reproduced with permission from the Royal College of Obstetricians and Gynaecologists).[4]

and plan management that considers all factors. If you have access to hysterosalpingography this can provide very valuable information.

> **Box 7.3:**   Case study
>
> Mr and Mrs Fallow attend your surgery to discuss their infertility tests that you had arranged when they had consulted you earlier, following 18 months of infertility at the ages of 37 and 39 years respectively. Although recent chlamydia swabs had been negative, in the past Mrs Fallow had been treated for a bout of serious pelvic inflammatory disease. In view of the risk of tubal disease, you arranged a hysterosalpingogram that revealed large bilateral hydrosalpinges. Her chlamydia serology is strongly positive but her other test results are unremarkable. Mr Fallow's external genitalia appear normal on examination and semen analysis is: volume 2.5 ml, pH 7.4, concentration 14 million per ml, motility 40% normal, morphology 4% normal forms.

Although hysterosalpingograms may suggest a tube is blocked when it is not in around 10% of cases, they are reliable at identifying hydrosalpinges. The prognosis for tubal surgery in this case is likely to be poor partly because of the unfavourable factors of large hydrosalpinges and chlamydia serology and because of the poor semen result (*see* Box 7.4 for normal values). Although the low borderline sperm count and reduced motility are of uncertain significance, the poor morphology suggests a poor prognosis. If these results were confirmed with a repeat semen test, the optimal treatment would be assisted conception using intracytoplasmic sperm injection (ICSI).

It is known that large hydrosalpinges reduce pregnancy rates and increase miscarriage rates. Thus salpingectomy, or at least occlusion of the proximal fallopian tubes, should be considered before proceeding with ICSI. The couple need referral for specialist care and if they proceed with ICSI treatment, they will need to be tested for hepatitis B and C and HIV to comply with the Human Fertilisation and Embryology Authority's (HFEA) guidelines on the storage of sperm and embryos.[7]

> **Box 7.4:**   World Health Organization normal semen analysis values[8]
> * Volume 2 ml or more
> * pH 7.2 or more
> * Sperm concentration >20 million per ml
> * Total sperm number 40 or more million sperm per ejaculate
> * Motility >50%
> * Morphology 15% or more normal forms
> * Sperm antibody tests:
>   - immunobead test <50% motile sperm bound to beads
>   - Mixed agglutination reaction (MAR) test <50% motile sperm bound

Male factor infertility

Around one in four infertile couples have evidence of male factor problems, and around one in 20 show a complete absence of any sperm. GPs should know how to manage the couple following the semen result particularly as the couple may become very distressed and even angry if the news is bad.

Box 7.5:   Case study

Mr and Mrs Baron have completed basic infertility investigations and have arranged an appointment with you to review their results. Mrs Baron has a cousin who has cystic fibrosis but she is a healthy 31 year old with no known medical problems. Mr Baron takes a beta blocker for hypertension, which is well controlled and he is otherwise well. The results of the investigations are given below.

Mrs Baron
- Rubella antibodies detected confirming immunity
- Luteinising hormone (LH) 3.1 IU/l Follicle stimulating hormone (FSH) 4 IU/l
- Progesterone 38 nmol/l
- Chlamydia serology negative

Mr Baron – semen analysis
- Volume 3.2 ml
- pH 7.2
- Liquefaction – normal
- No sperm were observed

At the initial consultation, you had not examined Mr Baron, but in view of the above discovery you now examine him. You discover that his testicles are small and he has a moderate sized varicocele on the left hand side. You are unable to positively identify his vas deferens on either side.

At the initial infertility consultation, you probably will not have adequate time for a complete assessment thus it is reasonable to defer the male genitalia examination until the result of the semen analysis is known. The main priority is to identify lumps that could be testicular cancer that necessitate urgent referral. Checking testicular volume and the presence of the vas deferens can provide very helpful information. If you are unfamiliar with this examination then it may be worth arranging to sit in on a clinic with a local specialist to learn more. There are conflicting views on the importance of varicoceles in male infertility, but the treatment of varicoceles is unlikely to be beneficial if the sperm count is very low.

Drugs may affect sperm production and/or ability to achieve intravaginal ejaculation. It is possible for beta blockers to cause impotence but they are not associated with azoospermia. As a first step, consult the *British National Formulary* (BNF) if you encounter a male problem with a man on medication.[9]

Azoospermia may be caused by chromosome abnormalities hence it is advisable to check his karyotype and also screen for Y deletions. The azoospermia could be caused by congenital bilateral absence of the vas deferens, which is associated with the carriage of cystic fibrosis mutations. In view of this genetic risk to the child, it is important to screen the couple for carriage of cystic fibrosis mutations.

The treatment options open to the couple are donor insemination and surgical sperm retrieval followed by ICSI. Both treatments are effective with pregnancy rates of 30% for one cycle of ICSI or about three cycles of donor insemination. Although if there is an obstructive cause for azoospermia it is usually possible to collect sperm surgically, if there are primary testicular problems then in many cases no sperm may be collected. A low testicular volume and blood tests such as follicle stimulating hormone (FSH) help predict the risk of not collecting sperm.

Ovulatory infertility

Irregular menstruation is a useful pointer to ovulatory dysfunction, which may be very responsive to appropriate treatment. However, to clarify the cause of irregular periods further tests are required beyond the basic investigations.

Box 7.6:   Case study

Mr and Mrs Nimble are a young couple who have completed basic infertility investigations. Mrs Nimble is a slim aerobics instructor who has erratic periods occurring at anything from 4 to 10 week intervals. In view of this, you had arranged a few additional tests and the results are given below.

- LH 14 IU/l
- FSH 4 IU/l
- Thyroid stimulating hormone (TSH) 2 nmol/l
- Prolactin 240 mU/l
- Sex hormone binding globulin (SHBG) 20 nmol/l
- Testosterone 3.2 nmol/l

The most common cause for irregular menstruation is polycystic ovarian syndrome (PCOS). This case has the typical biochemical features of a raised

LH, raised LH/FSH ratio (above 2.5), raised testosterone and lower SHBG levels. However, in many patients this is not the case and expert opinion is divided on the precise definition of PCOS, including the role and appearance of ultrasonography of the ovaries. Although hyperprolactinaemia is an infrequent cause of irregular menstruation, it is important to check prolactin levels, as one of the causes is pituitary microadenoma – hence specialist referral is appropriate.

The first step in the management of anovulatory PCOS is weight reduction if the woman is obese, but as with this patient not everyone with PCOS is obese. Opinion is divided regarding initial medication. First-line treatment used to be anti-oestrogen therapy with clomifene, but concerns about the risk of multiple pregnancies and ovarian cancer now make this approach less attractive. Insulin-sensitising agents such as metformin are used increasingly.

Box 7.7:   The public's views about the funding of infertility treatment

The science and discovery centre At-Bristol and the Centre for Reproductive Medicine, University of Bristol, surveyed visitors to the central shopping centre in Bristol and to the science centre website. Over 800 members of the public revealed overwhelming support for NHS funding of infertility services and an end to the 'post-code lottery' of provision. The survey showed that it was not generally felt that treatment should be denied solely due to a lower chance of success. However, the age of the mother was an important consideration with different views on what the upper age limit should be. NICE is expected to produce guidance on the availability of NHS funded treatment.[10]

Collecting data to demonstrate your learning, competence, performance and standards of service delivery: infertility

Example cycle of evidence 7.1

- Focus: clinical care

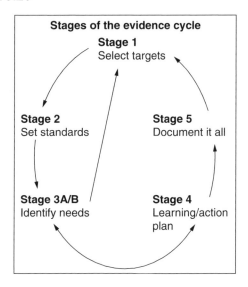

Stages of the evidence cycle

Stage 1
Select targets

Stage 2
Set standards

Stage 5
Document it all

Stage 3A/B
Identify needs

Stage 4
Learning/action plan

Box 7.8:   Case study

Mrs Lack visits your surgery at the start of her period to have a blood test for FSH and LH by your practice nurse for infertility assessment. She asks your practice nurse if the result of her husband's semen test is available yet. She has read an article on the Internet suggesting that she could improve her fertility by altering her diet. Your practice nurse discovers the semen test revealed a complete absence of sperm and pops her head around your door to ask what she should say to Mrs Lack.

As it would be a breach of confidentiality in respect of Mr Lack to give his wife his semen test result, you discuss the confidentiality issues with your practice nurse. Your practice nurse agrees that the results should be conveyed personally to Mr Lack with due sensitivity.

Checking the medical record you note the management plan is for the couple to return for a follow-up consultation to discuss the results when they are all available. Accordingly, you ask the practice nurse to check that such an appointment has been made and defer any discussion of results until then.

> This is just an example. Keep your task simple. You could choose three or four cycles of evidence to demonstrate your competence each year.

Stage 1: Select your aspirations for good practice

The excellent GP:

- keeps comprehensive records outlining the management plan and information given to patients including details of how results will be followed up and patients informed of results
- ensures that information is conveyed sensitively and appropriately respecting confidentiality.

Stage 2: Set the standards for your outcomes

Outcomes might include:

- the way learning is applied
- a learnt skill
- a protocol
- a strategy that is implemented
- meeting recommended standards.

- Demonstrate consistent best practice in providing assessment and treatment for infertile couples by checking that the last ten couples each had completed the basic tests outlined in RCOG guidelines.[4]
- Demonstrate consistent best practice in keeping good patient medical records, for instance by auditing the ten consultation records to see if the management plan was recorded at the end of each consultation.

Stage 3A: Identify your learning needs

- Consider if you know how to interpret the semen results that come from your local service, particularly considering what information you need to give to a patient depending on the result and what actions you should take.
- When recording data such as a semen analysis, undertake an audit that incorporates a check to review whether action is required such as checking that the patient has an appointment to discuss the result.

- Reflect on whether you know the current views on the link between diet and infertility.

Stage 3B: Identify your service needs

> Any of the needs assessment exercises in 3A may also reveal service needs.

- Track what happens to basic semen reports when received by the practice.
- Check whether the local laboratory follows WHO guidelines and the results they produce are consistent with WHO normal values.[4]
- Discuss with practice staff what information they give to patients about results of sensitive tests such as semen analysis.

Stage 4: Make and carry out a learning and action plan

- Read about semen tests, causes of abnormality and subsequent management options.
- Write up a simple handout for patients going through the significance of the results of the infertility tests you arrange, and discuss this with colleagues.
- Meet with the practice staff to talk through aspects of confidentiality of medical records. Consider producing (or updating) confidentiality guidelines for staff including reference to relevant resources such as: http://www.dataprotection.gov.uk/; http://www.gmc-uk.org.

Stage 5: Document your learning, competence, performance and standards of service delivery

- Keep track of all infertility consultations over a year and review how they were assessed and the patients informed of results.
- Discuss your approach to infertility with other health professionals and obtain their feedback.
- File your patient infertility results information sheet in your portfolio.

Box 7.9: Case study continued

Mr and Mrs Lack return to your surgery the following week, when you have had time to refresh yourself on the management of azoospermia and obtain all the test results. The couple were relieved that you gave them this news together and had a clear plan of action, starting with a repeat semen test for confirmation of the results. Having heard this news, they were less interested in the role of diet in infertility but were pleased that you were aware of the subject, providing them with simple advice and reassurance.

Example cycle of evidence 7.2

- Focus: maintaining good medical practice

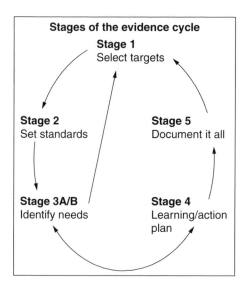

Stages of the evidence cycle

Stage 1
Select targets

Stage 2
Set standards

Stage 5
Document it all

Stage 3A/B
Identify needs

Stage 4
Learning/action plan

Box 7.10: Case study

Mrs Jumble presents to the surgery with irregular menstruation and for a repeat prescription of 'infertility tablets' (clomifene). Although she has been taking these for six months, her menstrual cycle remains irregular. Her mother had ovarian cancer and she has concerns that she may develop cancer herself. You notice she is a little overweight and perhaps slightly hirsute. She had been told that she has PCOS and she wonders if there may be a better treatment that she could try.

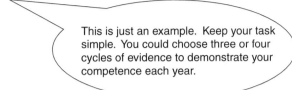

This is just an example. Keep your task simple. You could choose three or four cycles of evidence to demonstrate your competence each year.

Stage 1: Select your aspirations for good practice

The excellent GP:

- will be aware where to find best evidence on practice
- completes prescribing audits to ensure that patients do not continue treatment inappropriately.

Stage 2: Set the standards for your outcomes

Outcomes might include:

- the way learning is applied
- a learnt skill
- a protocol
- a strategy that is implemented
- meeting recommended standards.

- Demonstrate knowledge about best practice for the initial treatment options for ovulation induction in PCOS.
- Demonstrate best practice in the management of patients with PCOS.

Stage 3A: Identify your learning needs

- Discuss best current practice in the provision of insulin-sensitising agents such as metformin for treatment in PCOS with a GP with a special interest in sexual health. Realise some of what you didn't know previously.

Stage 3B: Identify your service needs

Any of the needs assessment exercises in 3A may also reveal service needs.

- Audit the use of clomifene in the practice and consider whether it has been monitored adequately and whether metformin may be a better alternative.
- Discuss the guidelines for the management of patients with infertility problems with relevant staff to determine whether any amendments are required.

Stage 4: Make and carry out a learning and action plan

- Perform a literature search for recent recommendations, especially any systematic reviews, for current best practice for treatment in PCOS.
- Obtain relevant guidelines e.g. from the RCOG. In this case, the RCOG provides useful guidelines on infertility,[4,11] the National electronic Library for Health provides access to Cochrane systematic reviews[6] and the *British National Formulary*[9] gives details about drugs. These resources will suggest metformin is regarded as an effective treatment for PCOS and that long-term use of clomifene may increase the risk of developing ovarian cancer. Additional advice will include the importance of losing weight and the small risk of lactic acidosis should the patient take metformin.

Stage 5: Document your learning, competence, performance and standards of service delivery

- Incorporate the new information in the guidelines for the use in your practice by all the clinicians.
- Re-audit the management of PCOS to confirm that the modern management guidelines are being followed.

Box 7.11:   Case study continued

Mrs Jumble presents three months later delighted that her menstrual cycle is now regular and she is optimistic that she may become pregnant.

Example cycle of evidence 7.3

- Focus: relationship[5] with patients

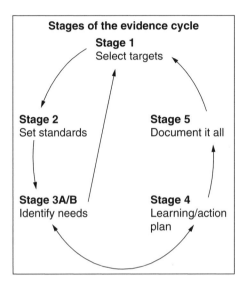

Stages of the evidence cycle

Stage 1
Select targets

Stage 2
Set standards

Stage 5
Document it all

Stage 3A/B
Identify needs

Stage 4
Learning/action plan

Box 7.12:   Case study

Mr and Mrs Lament attend your surgery to discuss their infertility tests. Her hysterosalpingogram revealed large bilateral hydrosalpinges and her husband has a low sperm count. You start to explain that they have serious barriers to a pregnancy and they may require assisted conception treatment. Mr Lament enquires whether there is anything he can do to improve his fertility. Mrs Lament wonders why she has developed tubal problems when she was never aware of any pelvic infection in the past. As the consultation progresses and you start to explain that it may be advisable to remove the fallopian tubes before considering assisted conception treatment Mrs Lament starts to cry.

This is just an example. Keep your task simple. You could choose three or four cycles of evidence to demonstrate your competence each year.

Stage 1: Select your aspirations for good practice

The excellent GP:

- provides patients with sufficient information to make choices about their management
- provides support for patients faced with difficult decisions and frustrations.

Stage 2: Set the standards for your outcomes

Outcomes might include:

- the way learning is applied
- a learnt skill
- a protocol
- a strategy that is implemented
- meeting recommended standards.

- Demonstrate best practice in providing information to patients.
- Develop your counselling skills through appropriate courses or through mentorship with a suitable peer or senior colleague.

Stage 3A: Identify your learning needs

- Self-assess your learning needs about breaking bad news – after an occasion when you had to do that.
- Complete a quiz in your GP newspaper about interpretation and results of infertility tests.

Stage 3B: Identify your service needs

Any of the needs assessment exercises in 3A may also reveal service needs.

- Get feedback from colleagues and staff for whom you are responsible, as to whether you recognise and are sensitive to patients' feelings and have strategies to deal with distressed patients.
- Conduct a 360° feedback exercise arranged by the practice team – focusing on breaking bad news and enabling patients to make informed decisions about treatment.

Stage 4: Make and carry out a learning and action plan

- Ask a colleague who has done a breaking bad news course to facilitate role play scenarios of difficult patient–staff interactions, where the patient is very distressed, at an in-house educational session for the team.
- Attend a course on breaking bad news.
- Sit in a clinic on one or more occasions with an infertility specialist and ask a myriad of questions about infertility tests and treatment.

Stage 5: Document your learning, competence, performance and standards of service delivery

- Keep records of interactions with other distressed patients and record your conclusions about your improvement in your reflective diary.
- Keep notes from attendance at the course.
- Retain copies of feedback from others in the team.

Box 7.13: Case study continued

You feel that you have identified the need for time in dealing with infertile couples when breaking bad news, and will consider how best to handle this in your surgery.

Example cycle of evidence 7.4

- Focus: working with colleagues
- Other relevant focus of evidence: teaching and training

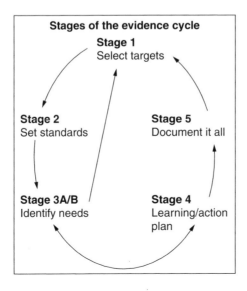

> **Box 7.14:** Case study
> A medical student is sitting in your surgery when a patient arrives asking for advice for infertility. The patient mentions that she has had a milky discharge from her breasts and has had no periods for four months.

> This is just an example. Keep your task simple. You could choose three or four cycles of evidence to demonstrate your competence each year.

Stage 1: Select your aspirations for good practice
The excellent GP:

- helps to educate other colleagues at all levels
- does not undermine the confidence of juniors or students.

Stage 2: Set the standards for your outcomes

> Outcomes might include:
>
> - the way learning is applied
> - a learnt skill
> - a protocol
> - a strategy that is implemented
> - meeting recommended standards.

- Demonstrate an active involvement in the training of another.

Stage 3A: Identify your learning needs
- Gain peer review of your teaching skills – ask another trainer to peer review a tutorial with the medical student.
- Self-assess your awareness of the curriculum of the local medical school.
- Check that your knowledge about galactorrhoea and amenorrhoea are up to date by comparing your performance with best practice guidelines.
- Feedback from trainees is a good way to assess your teaching, although it may be difficult to avoid bias if feedback is not anonymised.

- Check if you can answer questions posed by a medical student and if you have the skills to guide the student to solve the clinical problem, while taking care to ensure that the patient understands what he says.

Stage 3B: Identify your service needs

> Any of the needs assessment exercises in 3A may also reveal service needs.

- Undertake a force-field analysis with others in the practice team about the driving and restraining factors involved in practice teaching of medical students.

Stage 4: Make and carry out a learning and action plan

- Attend a meeting of the medical school curriculum group.
- Attend an update meeting about galactorrhoea and amenorrhoea and read widely about these subjects.
- Attend a 'training the trainers' course or if it is a while since you last went on a course, a refresher may be a good idea.
- Reflect on the outcome of force-field analysis with other teachers in the practice. Make plan to boost driving factors.

Stage 5: Document your learning, competence, performance and standards of service delivery

- Keep feedback from the medical student.
- Record outcome of force-field analysis.
- Download notes about galactorrhoea from a professional body.
- Keep completed quiz with right answers where relevant.

Box 7.15: Case study continued

At the end of the consultation, the patient feels happy that her condition has been explained so thoroughly and feels confident that a knowledgeable doctor is managing her. The medical student is grateful for the opportunity to learn about galactorrhoea and amenorrhoea with a real clinical perspective.

References

1   Jenkins JM, Corrigan L and Chambers R (2002) *Infertility Matters in Healthcare.* Radcliffe Medical Press, Oxford.

2   Collins JA, Burrows EA and Willan AR (1995) The prognosis for live birth among untreated infertile couples. *Fertil Steril.* **64**: 22–8.

3   www.repromed.org.uk/book/content/Fertility_Calculator.htm.

4   Royal College of Obstetricians and Gynaecologists (1998) *The Initial Investigation and Management of the Infertile Couple. National evidence-based clinical guidelines.* Royal College of Obstetricians and Gynaecologists, London. www.rcog.org.uk/guidelines.asp=1088GuidelineID=25.

5   Cahill DJ and Wardle PG (2002) Management of infertility. *BMJ.* **325**: 28–32. http://bmj.com/cgi/content/full/325/7354/28?maxtoshow=.

6   www.nelh.nhs.uk.

7   Human Fertilisation and Embryology Authority (2001) *Screening of Patients. Letter 6th June 2001 from HFEA Chairman to all IVF clinics.* HFEA, London.

8   World Health Organization (1999) *WHO Laboratory Manual for the Examination of Human Semen and Sperm–Cervical Mucus Interaction* (4e). Cambridge University Press, Cambridge.

9   Joint Formulary Committee (2003) *British National Formulary.* British Medical Association and Royal Pharmaceutical Society of Great Britain, London. www.bnf.org.

10 http://www.bionews.org.uk/commentary.lasso?storyid=1719.

11 www.rcog.org.uk.

8

Vaginal bleeding problems in general practice

There are many vaginal bleeding problems that may lead a woman to see her GP. This chapter will focus on some of the more common bleeding problems related to menstruation and early pregnancy providing references to more in-depth information available on the Internet.

What issues you should cover

Menorrhagia

Box 8.1: Case study

Mrs Flud is a 43 year old woman who attends your surgery distraught that over the last five months her periods have become increasingly heavy and trouble-some. Her menstrual cycle remains regular and she had a normal cervical smear six months earlier. She feels tired all the time and is fed up with her heavy periods. However, she does not want a hysterectomy and she is concerned that if she seeks medical help from the hospital she will be forced to lose her uterus.

Before considering treatment, it is important to consider whether there may be any significant underlying pathology. The Royal College of Obstetricians and Gynaecologists (RCOG) provides helpful guidelines on the initial manage-ment of menorrhagia, which are summarised in Figure 8.1. The full guidelines may be viewed by visiting the RCOG website.[1] If, following examination, you find that Mrs Flud has no obvious worrying features you can next consider treatment options.

A study of a cohort of women in Oxford up to the end of 1989 suggested that around one in five women in the UK had had a hysterectomy before 55 years of age.[2] In many of these cases the uterus was normal, particularly

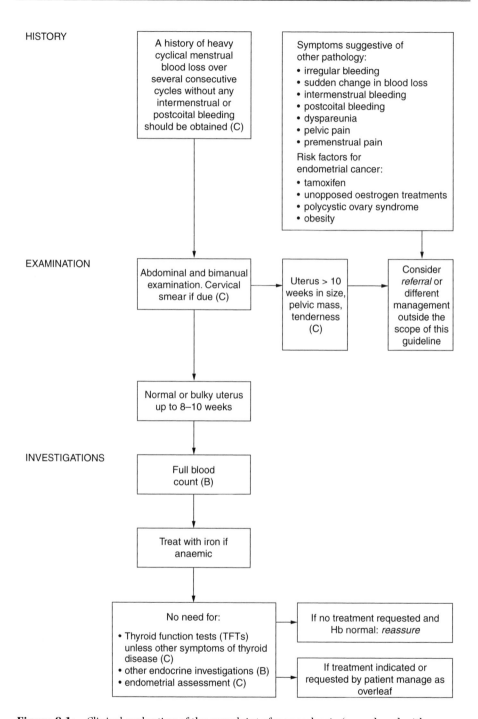

HISTORY

A history of heavy cyclical menstrual blood loss over several consecutive cycles without any intermenstrual or postcoital bleeding should be obtained (C)

Symptoms suggestive of other pathology:
• irregular bleeding
• sudden change in blood loss
• intermenstrual bleeding
• postcoital bleeding
• dyspareunia
• pelvic pain
• premenstrual pain

Risk factors for endometrial cancer:
• tamoxifen
• unopposed oestrogen treatments
• polycystic ovary syndrome
• obesity

EXAMINATION

Abdominal and bimanual examination. Cervical smear if due (C)

Uterus > 10 weeks in size, pelvic mass, tenderness (C)

Consider *referral* or different management outside the scope of this guideline

Normal or bulky uterus up to 8–10 weeks

INVESTIGATIONS

Full blood count (B)

Treat with iron if anaemic

No need for:
• Thyroid function tests (TFTs) unless other symptoms of thyroid disease (C)
• other endocrine investigations (B)
• endometrial assessment (C)

If no treatment requested and Hb normal: *reassure*

If treatment indicated or requested by patient manage as overleaf

Figure 8.1:   Clinical evaluation of the complaint of menorrhagia (reproduced with permission from the Royal College of Obstetricians and Gynaecologists).[1] Level of evidence: (A), based on randomised controlled trials; (B), based on other robust experimental or observational studies; (C), based on more limited evidence but the advice relies on expert opinion and has the endorsement of respected authorities.

in parous women. However, improvements in conservative management of menorrhagia provide many options to improve Mrs Flud's heavy periods without a hysterectomy[3] and the RCOG provides guidelines for medical management in primary care (*see* Figure 8.2). The levonorgestrel intrauterine system (IUS) is a good method that has been shown to produce up to a 90% reduction in menstrual loss.[4] The IUS also reduces dysmenorrhoea and provides contraception[5] (*see* Chapter 5 for further details).

Even if medical therapy is unsuccessful there are several new techniques to ablate the endometrium without removing the uterus, producing satisfactory results in 80–90% of patients.[6] Check on the local availability and gynaecologists' experience with new techniques such as balloon systems delivering local heat in the uterus, devices delivering radiofrequency thermal energy or electromagnetic energy in the uterine cavity and endometrial cryoablation. Even if Mrs Flud has symptomatic fibroids, uterine artery embolisation conserving the uterus has been shown to provide a satisfactory result in around 90% of cases.[7]

Box 8.2:   Case study continued

Mrs Flud has no indicators of serious pathology but a full blood count shows that she is mildly iron deficient and she starts taking some oral iron. After discussion of the options, she decides to have a levonorgestrel intrauterine system fitted. She needs support to continue with it as her menstrual loss is not immediately improved but after six months of use she is pleased to find that her periods are much more manageable.

Dysmenorrhoea and endometriosis

Box 8.3:   Case study

Following a particularly painful period, 22-year-old Miss Payne visits your surgery complaining that she is unable to cope with the pain any longer. Over the last few months she has found that simple analgesia has become progressively less effective, although she was relieved that between her periods she had no significant discomfort. Although not in a relationship at present, she wishes to have children in the future, and she is concerned that her elder sister has recently had a total abdominal hysterectomy and bilateral salpingoophorectomy for endometriosis.

Although it is not possible to make a definitive diagnosis of endometriosis without visualising it, usually by laparoscopy for pelvic deposits or ultrasonography

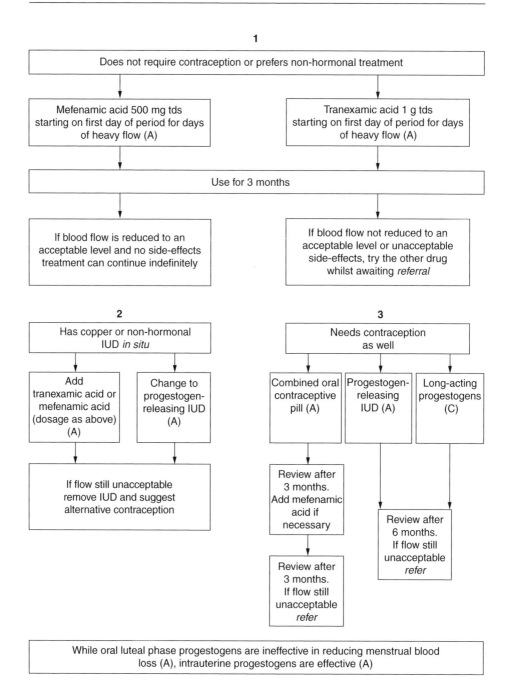

Figure 8.2: Medical management of the complaint of menorrhagia (reproduced with permission from the Royal College of Obstetricians and Gynaecologists).[1] This figure outlines different approaches to treatment depending on whether the patient does not require contraception (1), is using non-hormonal contraception (2) or requires contraception (3). Evidence levels (A), (B) and (C) are the same as in Figure 8.1.

for endometriomas, the above history is highly suggestive. Nevertheless, it would be inappropriate to label the patient as having endometriosis without investigation. Consider alternative diagnoses such as idiopathic dysmenorrhoea, irritable bowel syndrome and pelvic inflammatory disease. Ask her about her bowels and symptoms of infection. Vaginal examination may uncover significant tenderness if there are endometriotic deposits present or an enlarged ovary if it contains an endometrioma. If a woman is not trying to conceive and vaginal examination reveals no abnormality, symptomatic relief may be attempted using the combined oral contraceptive pill (monthly or tricycling by taking three packets sequentially without a break) with non-steroidal anti-inflammatory drugs during her periods.

However, if the pain is not controlled by this treatment, or if the patient is anxious, then it would be appropriate to refer her to a gynaecologist for a laparoscopy to establish the diagnosis. Endometriosis may be controlled by progestogens, danazol or gonadotrophin releasing hormone (GnRH) agonists (with add back oestrogen therapy if prolonged). Surgical treatment by ablation or excision laparoscopically or at laparotomy may prove necessary for control of the pain.[8] Further information on the investigation and management of endometriosis can be found on the RCOG website.[9]

Box 8.4:   Case study continued

Miss Payne returns after taking three packs of a combined oral contraceptive and is obviously unhappy. Despite an improvement in the pain, she is still very anxious that her future fertility will be affected, so you agree to refer her to a specialist.

Threatened miscarriage of pregnancy

Box 8.5:   Case study

Following an anxious night, Mrs Loss attends your surgery as soon as it opens. She has had light vaginal bleeding but no pain at eight weeks' gestation in her second pregnancy. In her first pregnancy she had miscarried at seven weeks and she is very concerned that she may miscarry again. She has read on the Internet that progesterone may prevent miscarriages and she is desperate to do anything to save her pregnancy.

The main concern about this patient is about the viability of the pregnancy, so it is appropriate to arrange an urgent pelvic ultrasound scan. This can also exclude the less likely, but very serious, possibility that she may have an ectopic pregnancy. Most parts of the UK can provide same day access to an early pregnancy assessment unit (EPAU) that can provide emergency ultrasound scans and assist in patient management. If a same day scan can be performed then a vaginal examination is unlikely to contribute to management and a sympathetic approach to the patient is very important, avoiding unnecessary examinations. The RCOG website provides more detailed guidance on the management of early pregnancy loss.[10]

Although it is very tempting to agree to patients' requests for treatments that may not cause harm, the current RCOG guidelines recommend that the value of progesterone to reduce the risk of recurrent miscarriage remains unproven. At present progesterone should only be used in this condition in the context of research studies.

Recurrent miscarriage is defined as the loss of at least three pregnancies and affects 1 in 100 women. Couples may be distraught after two miscarriages, particularly if associated with infertility and increased female age. Some treatments are controversial and assessment of patients may differ between colleagues. This is a good topic for training and development of shared guidelines that are acceptable to all your colleagues in primary and secondary care. The RCOG guidelines provide a good starting point for you to use.[11]

Box 8.6: Case study continued

Mrs Loss attends a week later having had a scan that shows that she has a viable pregnancy. She wants to discuss whether she should stop her work as a secretary now to avoid any further risk to the pregnancy. You have read through the guidelines and are able to go through them with her. Although she has to decide for herself whether her anxiety merits stopping work, you advise her that normal activities are unlikely to make any difference to her risk of miscarriage.

Suspected ectopic pregnancy

Box 8.7: Case study

Following your morning surgery, you visit Mrs Burst, who had called earlier complaining of severe lower abdominal pain. When you arrive, the pain has settled a little after she had taken paracetamol. Her last period had started two days earlier, but had been 12 days late and was light even though she had an IUCD *in situ*. However, her periods have always tended to be irregular so Mrs Burst had thought nothing of this. Abdominal examination revealed lower abdominal tenderness and mild pyrexia.

Although the diagnosis is unclear, it is sensible to arrange emergency admission as she may have an ectopic pregnancy on the threshold of rupture. In view of the possibility of appendicitis or other surgical pathology, there is a dilemma as to whether to admit her to a gynaecological ward or a surgical ward. If you carry a sensitive pregnancy test urine dipstick with you, you may resolve this dilemma. If the pregnancy test is positive, then gynaecological admission is appropriate, whereas if the test is negative you may need to think further. Although abdominal examination can prove very useful, vaginal examination is a risky examination to perform at the patient's home especially without a chaperone and you should consider whether this examination will alter your management.

If you have decided to admit the patient, the decision then rests between surgical or gynaecological admission. The history and abdominal examination will generally steer you in the right direction for initial referral, and gynaecologists and surgeons can refer to each other. The differential diagnosis includes other gynaecological problems such as complications from ovarian cysts and acute pelvic inflammatory disease, for which the RCOG provides guidelines on management.[12]

When arranging admission it is useful to establish if she has been seen in the hospital previously. It is all too easy to generate duplicate medical records when patients are admitted without checking for previous records. This can lead to later problems when searching for information about the patient.

Box 8.8:   Case study continued

You stay with Mrs Burst until the ambulance arrives, in case her condition deteriorates acutely, if an ectopic pregnancy were to rupture. You check her blood pressure and pulse and ensure that the patient is handed over to the ambulance staff before you leave her.

Amenorrhoea

Comprehensive guidance on the management of amenorrhoea in general practice is available from Prodigy.[13]

Box 8.9:   Case study

Miss Little attends with her mother who does all the talking. Her mother says she is worried as her daughter, who has just had her 15th birthday, has not yet had a period.

What issues you should cover

If this information is not volunteered you may need to ask specifically about the following points.

- Establish with Miss Little that her mother does mean that she has *never* had a period, not just none for two months! It is possible, too, for ovulation to occur prior to a first period. Always think about pregnancy.
- Find out the age when the mother and any sisters started their periods, as it may be constitutional. That is, the pulsatile production of GnRH occurs later in some families.
- Determine if there is any family history of any genetic disorders such as Turner's syndrome (if it is mild with only short stature and web neck it may escape notice until puberty).
- Chronic illness, weight loss, anorexia, high levels of exercise or stress can cause hypothalamic dysfunction. Breast milk production might suggest prolactin excess.
- Cyclical abdominal pain may suggest a genitourinary abnormality such as an imperforate hymen or an absent vagina with a functioning uterus.
- Enquire if there has been previous treatment e.g. with chemotherapy, as you may not know about previous treatment for a brain tumour, or for a hydrocephalus.

The examination

Check her weight and height to establish her BMI. If the BMI is less than 19, regular menstruation is unlikely. Ask Miss Little if she would like a chaperone for any examination. She may prefer to have a nurse present, rather than her mother, and this gives you another opportunity to check the history (e.g. about risk of pregnancy or anorexia) from her. Chart the secondary sexual characteristics (*see* Table 8.1). Look for signs of hypothyroidism, hirsutes, and features of Turner's syndrome. If she consents to you looking at her external genitalia, record your findings, but pelvic examination is not useful or appropriate at this stage.

Investigations

If she has secondary sexual characteristics and you are at all suspicious, do a pregnancy test.

Primary amenorrhoea is defined as the failure to establish menstruation by the age of 14 years if there are no signs of secondary sexual maturation, or by the age of 16 years if normal secondary sexual characteristics are developing.[15] Refer for further investigations if a patient falls into either of these categories.

Table 8.1:   Tanner's stages of puberty in females[14]

Stage	Breast	Pubic hair
1: Pre-adolescent	Only papillae are elevated.	Vellus hair only and hair is similar to development over anterior abdominal wall (i.e. no pubic hair).
2	Breast bud and papilla are elevated and a small mount is present; areola diameter is enlarged.	There is sparse growth of long, slightly pigmented, downy hair or only slightly curled hair, appearing along labia.
3	Further enlargement of breast mound; increased palpable glandular tissue.	Hair is darker, coarser, more curled, and spreads to the pubic junction.
4	Areola and papilla are elevated to form a second mound above the level of the rest of the breast.	Adult-type hair; area covered is less than that in most adults; there is no spread to the medial surface of thighs.
5: Adult	Adult mature breast; recession of areola to the mound of breast tissue, rounding of the breast mound, and projection of only the papillae are evident.	Adult-type hair with increased spread to medial surface of thighs; distribution is as an inverse triangle.

Box 8.10:   Case study continued

Miss Little has some secondary sexual characteristics equivalent, you think, to stage 3. Both she and her mother are small and thin and her BMI is only 19. You discuss with her about avoiding smoking and having a good diet. You advise her to increase her calcium intake, how to ensure that she has sufficient sunlight for vitamin D production and to take plenty of weight bearing exercise to maximise her bone mass. You arrange to see her again in six months if she has not started her periods, or before then if any new symptoms appear.

Secondary amenorrhoea

Box 8.11: Case study

Mrs Reed, a miserable looking thin woman of 39 years, normally attends one of your partners quite frequently with multiple somatic complaints, so you are a little wary. She tells you that the practice nurse suggested that she consulted you as she has not had a proper period for months and is feeling terrible. On enquiry, you eventually determine that her last episode of bleeding was about eight or nine weeks ago and she complained to your partner about how heavy it was at the time, but she has not had a regular cycle for years.

What issues you should cover

Exclude pregnancy with a pregnancy test. It may seem obvious, but check that she is not receiving a progestogen-only method of contraception (*see* Chapter 5) that would give her irregular periods.

You would usually wait until six months of amenorrhoea until putting in train other investigations, but you might have a lower threshold for investigations in this chronically unwell woman.

As in primary amenorrhoea, chronic illness or stress can cause hypothalamic dysfunction. She may have problems arising from weight loss or anorexia or possibly high levels of exercise, in which case you should enquire regarding visual disturbance. Breast milk production might suggest prolactin excess. Avoid examining the breasts for expression of milk if you are going to take blood for a prolactin level as it may raise the level. Ask about symptoms suggestive of thyroid disease. Check that she is not taking any antipsychotic or other medication that might affect hypothalamic function. Look out for symptoms or signs that would suggest PCOS which occurs in 30% of women with secondary amenorrhoea.[16] Not all patients with PCOS have obesity with hyperpigmentation of the skin folds, but she might have excess body hair, alopecia, acne and a history of difficulty with conception. She might have similar symptoms and signs with rarer conditions like Cushing's syndrome or, if excess body hair has developed rapidly, adrenal hyperplasia, an adrenal tumour or an ovarian androgen-producing tumour.

Symptoms of hot flushes might suggest premature ovarian failure (*see* Chapter 9) and may be associated with autoimmune conditions such as hypothyroidism, diabetes or Addison's disease. Occasionally structural abnormalities of the vagina, stenosis of the cervix or adhesions in the uterus can cause amenorrhoea, usually with complaints of abdominal pain.

Choosing your investigations

Always do a pregnancy test. Take blood for the levels of FSH, LH, prolactin (*see* Table 8.2 for interpretation in common conditions) and thyroid function in all patients with secondary amenorrhoea. Testosterone levels may be useful in patients with hirsutes. If the levels of testosterone are in the male range, an adrenal or androgenic tumour may be present prompting specialist referral.

Oestradiol blood levels vary too much to be useful, but a progestogen challenge test can show that adequate oestrogens are present. Do not use this test if you suspect any structural obstruction to the menstrual flow. If you give medroxyprogesterone acetate 10 mg once a day for seven days, a withdrawal bleed will follow unless oestradiol levels are low.

Pelvic ultrasound may show the classic picture of polycystic ovaries with their string of pearls appearance from the multiple small peripherally situated cysts.

Table 8.2: Hormone results in common causes of amenorrhoea

	FSH	LH	Prolactin	Testosterone
Hyperprolactinaemia (requires further investigation regarding cause)	Normal or low	Normal or low	High	Normal
Polycystic ovarian syndrome	Normal	Normal or slightly raised	Normal or moderate rise	Slightly raised
Premature menopause	Very high	High	Normal	Normal
Hypothalamic e.g. with weight loss, excess exercise, stress	Normal or low	Normal or low	Normal	Normal

If you are still uncertain about the underlying cause, or about how to manage a condition you have identified, you might wish to refer to a gynaecologist. A patient with a high prolactin will require computerised tomography (CT) or magnetic resonance imaging (MRI) and specialist advice from an endocrinologist.

Correction of underlying causes such as anorexia may require referral to a psychologist or psychiatrist, but lesser degrees of weight loss or over-exercising can be managed in general practice.

PCOS responds best to weight loss. Patients often require treatment for associated lipid disorders, diabetes or hypertension. Treatment with metformin may be considered but evidence for prevention of long-term adverse outcomes is not yet available. You could consult the management guidance of the RCOG.[17]

Box 8.12:   Case study continued

Mrs Reed's investigations are all normal except for a slightly raised prolactin level. You tell her that her tests do not suggest that she is menopausal as she assumed. You suggest that she keeps a record of her menstrual loss over the next six months. Later in the year, your partner tells you that she has moved onto other complaints and has not mentioned her periods again!

Collecting data to demonstrate your learning, competence, performance and standards of service delivery: vaginal bleeding problems

Example cycle of evidence 8.1

- Focus: clinical care
- Other relevant focus of evidence: maintaining good medical practice

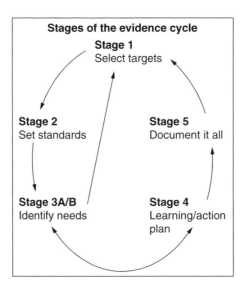

Stages of the evidence cycle

Stage 1
Select targets

Stage 2
Set standards

Stage 5
Document it all

Stage 3A/B
Identify needs

Stage 4
Learning/action plan

Box 8.13: Case study

Mrs Razor presents to your surgery troubled that her periods have become irregular. She is unhappy with her body image and she wishes to lose weight, which has been gradually increasing since her 40th birthday last year. She now weighs 90 kg at a height of 1.65 m. As you discuss her problems, it becomes apparent that there is something that is causing her worry and embarrassment. Eventually she summons the courage to tell you that her main problem is that she has more frequently needed to shave her legs, and she is worried that she is becoming more 'hairy'.

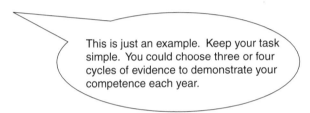

This is just an example. Keep your task simple. You could choose three or four cycles of evidence to demonstrate your competence each year.

Stage 1: Select your aspirations for good practice

The excellent GP:

- is sympathetic to the concerns of patients and recognises the presenting complaint may not always be the main concern
- provides patients with the opportunity and the confidence to discuss sensitive issues.

Stage 2: Set the standards for your outcomes

Outcomes might include:

- the way learning is applied
- a learnt skill
- a protocol
- a strategy that is implemented
- meeting recommended standards.

- Demonstrable consistent best practice in management of PCOS and related problems.
- Enthusiasm to address weight problems for patients who consult with obesity.

Stage 3A: Identify your learning needs

- Self-assess and reflect on your own learning needs in respect of PCOS with regard to diagnosis and management.
- Significant event audit of delayed diagnosis in the case of PCOS.

Stage 3B: Identify your service needs

> Any of the needs assessment exercises in 3A may also reveal service needs.

- Review the advice provided by your practice to obese individuals who wish to lose weight – how does it compare against national guidelines?
- Audit the records of patients with important co-morbidities such as diabetes mellitus and hypertension to see if appropriate advice about diet and their weight has been given to these patients.

Stage 4: Make and carry out a learning and action plan

- The RCOG provide guidelines on the long-term consequences of PCOS, which may provide a useful update on this condition.[17]
- As there are many controversial aspects regarding PCOS you may find it useful to discuss this condition with a local gynaecology specialist or attend a lecture on the subject where you can discuss your queries.
- Arrange a presentation in your practice by yourself or an invited speaker to discuss the implications and management of obesity and PCOS.

Stage 5: Document your learning, competence, performance and standards of service delivery

- Write your own notes about the recognition and management of PCOS and keep a record of key references including useful website pages in your learning portfolio.
- For later reference make a note of the development webpage for NICE guidelines on 'Obesity: the prevention, identification, evaluation, treatment and weight maintenance of overweight and obesity in adults'.[18]

Box 8.14: Case study continued

Following confirmation of the diagnosis of PCOS by ultrasound scan and slight elevation of serum androgens, Mrs Razor was relieved to hear your explanation of her symptoms. Recognising the importance of weight reduction, Mrs Razor had altered her lifestyle to increase the amount of exercise and was now on a long-term diet plan aiming for gradual but sustained weight reduction.

Example cycle of evidence 8.2

- Focus: relationships with patients

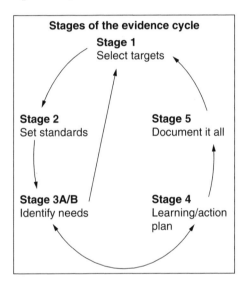

Stages of the evidence cycle

Stage 1 Select targets

Stage 2 Set standards

Stage 3A/B Identify needs

Stage 4 Learning/action plan

Stage 5 Document it all

Box 8.15: Case study

Mrs Weeds is a 63-year-old widow, who attends your surgery anxious to report that she had started to bleed vaginally.

This is just an example. Keep your task simple. You could choose three or four cycles of evidence to demonstrate your competence each year.

Stage 1: Select your aspirations for good practice
The excellent GP:

• will support patients at times of particular stress such as around the time of possible detection of cancer
• will be aware when a minor symptom may indicate the possibility of a serious condition and convey this information to patients.

Stage 2: Set the standards for your outcomes

Outcomes might include:

• the way learning is applied
• a learnt skill
• a protocol
• a strategy that is implemented
• meeting recommended standards.

• Establishment of appropriate patient education and screening processes in place to detect gynaecological cancers at early stage.

Stage 3A: Identify your learning needs
• Consider what you know and what patients should know about endometrial cancer, cervical cancer, ovarian cancer and vulval cancer.
• Compare contents and diagnoses in response letters from consultants to whom you have referred patients with contents and assumed diagnoses in your initial referral letters.
• Self-assess if you are able to inform patients of what symptoms and signs to look out for without causing alarm. Invite retrospective feedback from patients.

Stage 3B: Identify your service needs

Any of the needs assessment exercises in 3A may also reveal service needs.

• Review the quantity and quality of patient information sources e.g. leaflets and websites for gynaecological cancer and self-assess yours and colleagues' knowledge and skills.

- Find out the latest figures on the availability and accessibility of investigations and treatment for a variety of gynaecological cancers.

Stage 4: Make and carry out a learning and action plan

- Ensure that you are aware of current best practice in screening and initial management of gynaecological cancers by reading, discussion with colleagues and attending an update lecture or workshop.
- Obtain and study the referral protocol for signs and symptoms that might be construed as those of gynaecological cancers.

Stage 5: Document your learning, competence, performance and standards of service delivery

- Although verbal praise (as below) is very satisfying, a written statement could form valuable evidence for your portfolio. You could ask the patient to drop you a line after viewing the website material so that you could know whether to recommend this site to other patients and provide you with a written record of the patient's views.
- Keep notes from your learning plan.

Box 8.16:   Case study continued

Two weeks later Mrs Weeds returns to your surgery with her daughter. She has had an ultrasound scan and outpatient hysteroscopy, which confirmed a diagnosis of endometrial cancer. The hospital consultant had explained what this meant and arranged for her to be admitted shortly for a hysterectomy. However, she could not remember everything that was said, hence her daughter wondered if there was any website they could access for information to read at their own pace. The patient was pleased with your sympathetic management when she initially presented and was delighted that you were able to point them to the CancerBACUP website.[19]

Example cycle of evidence 8.3

- Focus: working with colleagues
- Other relevant foci of evidence: teaching and training

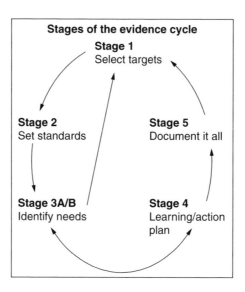

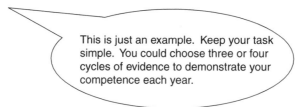

Box 8.17:   Case study

You are leading on infertility management for your team and are drafting guidelines for recurrent miscarriage for the practice with the help of the local hospital infertility consultant.

This is just an example. Keep your task simple. You could choose three or four cycles of evidence to demonstrate your competence each year.

Stage 1: Select your aspirations for good practice

The excellent GP:

- respects the views of colleagues and patients when developing group guidelines on best practice
- helps to train professional colleagues and share knowledge.

Stage 2: Set the standards for your outcomes

Outcomes might include:

- the way learning is applied
- a learnt skill
- a protocol
- a strategy that is implemented
- meeting recommended standards.

- Develop practice guidelines for management of recurrent miscarriage, considering the availability of local resources and local opinion and best practice from national guidelines.[11]

Stage 3A: Identify your learning needs

- Review your knowledge of recurrent miscarriage and the costs of investigations.
- Review the significance and interpretation of tests such as for thrombophilia and antiphospholipid screening.

Stage 3B: Identify your service needs

Any of the needs assessment exercises in 3A may also reveal service needs.

- Assess current practice by reviewing the investigations, ease of referral or admission of the last few patients presenting with recurrent miscarriage.

Stage 4: Make and carry out a learning and action plan

- Arrange a visit to your practice from a local specialist, preferably from a local recurrent miscarriage clinic if you have one. Invite others to join in from across your PCO to discuss local guidelines.
- Discuss management with colleagues and draft, then agree, consensus guidelines.

Stage 5: Document your learning, competence, performance and standards of service delivery

- Document brief minutes of meetings to produce guidelines for inclusion in your portfolio with a copy of the final guidelines.

Box 8.18:   Case study continued

You find that drafting guidelines for your practice or the local area is a good educational process that encourages working effectively with your colleagues.

References

1   http://www.rcog.org.uk/guidelines.asp?PageID=108&GuidelineID=28.

2   Vessey M, Villard L, Mackintosh M *et al.* (1992) The epidemiology of hysterectomy: findings in a large cohort study. *Br J Obstet Gynaecol.* **99**: 402–7.

3   Porteous A and Prentice A (2003) Medical management of dysfunctional uterine bleeding. *Reviews in Gynaecological Practice.* **3**: 81–4.

4   Lethaby A, Cooke I and Rees M (2002) *Progesterone/progestogen Releasing Intra-uterine System for Heavy Menstrual Bleeding* (Cochrane Review). The Cochrane Library, issue 4. Update Software, Oxford.

5   Barrington JW and Bowen-Simpkins P (1997) The levonorgestrel intrauterine system in the management of menorrhagia. *Br J Obstet Gynaecol.* **104**: 614–16.

6   Sowter MC (2003) New surgical treatments for menorrhagia. *Lancet.* **361**: 1456–8.

7   Pron G, Bennett J, Common A *et al.* and Ontario Uterine Fibroid Embolization Collaborative Group (2003) The Ontario Uterine Fibroid Embolization Trial. Part 2. Uterine fibroid reduction and symptom relief after uterine artery embolization for fibroids. *Fertil Steril.* **79**: 120–7.

8   Winkel CA (2003) Evaluation and management of women with endometriosis. *Obstet & Gynecol.* **102**: 397–408.

9   http://www.rcog.org.uk/guidelines.asp?PageID=106&GuidelineID=10.

10   http://www.rcog.org.uk/guidelines.asp?PageID=106&GuidelineID=8.

11   http://www.rcog.org.uk/guidelines.asp?PageID=106&GuidelineID=46.

12   http://www.rcog.org.uk/guidelines.asp?PageID=106&GuidelineID=49.

13   http://www.prodigy.nhs.uk/guidance.asp?gt=Amenorrhoea.

14   Marshall WA and Tanner JM (1969) Variations in pattern of pubertal changes in girls. *Arch Dis Child.* **44(235)**: 291–303.

15 Edmonds DK (ed.) (1999) *Dewhurst's Textbook of Obstetrics and Gynaecology for Postgraduates* (6e). Blackwell Science, Oxford.

16 Hopkinson ZE, Sattar N, Fleming R and Greer IA (1998) Polycystic ovarian syndrome: the metabolic syndrome comes to gynaecology. *BMJ.* **317**: 329–32.

17 http://www.rcog.org.uk/guidelines.asp?PageID=106&GuidelineID=50.

18 http://www.nice.org.uk.

19 http://www.cancerbacup.org.uk/info/womb.htm.

9

The menopause

Box 9.1: Case study

A woman recently registered with your general practice attends asking if she could be 'on the change'.

What issues you should cover

Age

Usually the menopause happens between the ages of 48 and 54 years, but it may occur outside these ages. The median age of menopause is 51 years old. The *menopause* is the permanent stopping of menstruation resulting from loss of ovarian follicle activity. The natural menopause is defined as being after 12 months of no menstruation, so can only be decided after the event.

The *perimenopause* includes the time beginning with the first features of the approaching menopause, such as hot flushes or menstrual irregularity. It ends 12 months after the last menstrual period. The *postmenopause* starts with the last menstrual period but cannot be dated with certainty until 12 months have occurred without menstruation.

A *premature menopause* is usually defined as the permanent cessation of menstrual periods due to loss of ovarian follicular activity occurring before 40 years of age. A *surgical menopause* occurs when the ovaries are removed. This is sometimes done together with a hysterectomy and causes a sudden drop in female hormone level, often with severe symptoms.

Timing of her last period

She could be having menopausal symptoms even if she is still having menstrual periods (perimenopause) but you would also want to think about alternative reasons for hot sweats (e.g. anxiety, pyrexia) or psychological symptoms (e.g. worsening premenstrual syndrome or depression).[1]

If she has not had a recent period, ensure that she is not pregnant. Many women think that they cannot become pregnant if they are coming up to 50 years of age and stop using contraception. If she is at risk of pregnancy, arrange a pregnancy test and discuss contraceptive precautions with her.[2]

If she has been having periods, she may be worried because she has missed periods or had them more frequently and that the amount of loss is different. Periods may become closer together when ovulation is not occurring because the luteal phase is shortened. The luteal phase occurs after ovulation when the corpus luteum, formed from the cells around the released ovum, produces progesterone to maintain the endometrium ready for a fertilised ovum. Irregular loss of the endometrium occurs when insufficient progesterone is produced. This loss is light or absent if oestrogen levels are also lowered. The loss can be heavy if oestrogen levels are fluctuating and sometimes high enough to increase the thickness of the endometrium.

Hot flushes

If she has been having hot flushes establish how often they are occurring, how much of a nuisance they are and whether they are disturbing her sleep. Being woken several times a night can lead to irritability and loss of concentration the following day, especially if she has to get out of bed to change nightwear or sheets because of sweating.

Vaginal dryness

Thinning of the vaginal walls, less lubrication and discomfort with sexual intercourse tend to occur after several years of lowered hormone levels but some women will develop this earlier. Many women will not volunteer this information but will be grateful for a chance to discuss it.

Formication

You may also need to ask about this condition of feeling as if something is crawling just under the skin, as many women do not like to mention it. They often think that it is a sign of a psychiatric illness and are very reassured to discover that it can occur as a symptom of the menopause.

Bladder symptoms

Urgency and frequency of micturition are often associated with vaginal dryness and she may have noticed a tendency to have more frequent urinary tract infections. Incontinence or difficulties passing urine are more likely to be associated with structural abnormalities such as urogenital prolapse.

Psychological symptoms

There is no clear evidence that changes in hormone levels at the menopause can cause depression and most women do not have major mood changes around their menopause.[3] The physical changes of the menopause may make it more difficult to cope with the many major life stresses that occur in 40–60 year olds of both sexes. If psychological symptoms are prominent, enquire about other stressful events such as:

• parents ageing and becoming dependent
• deaths of family or friends
• loss of partner through death, separation or divorce
• children leaving home
• demanding workload
• family worries such as partner's job, children's marriages, etc.
• poor health
• money worries
• coming to terms with her own ageing.

Worries about osteoporosis[4,5]

If she is concerned about having thinning of her bones, establish if this is because she has symptoms of aching or swelling of her joints. Symptoms will need independent evaluation for their cause but are often part of the ageing process rather than being due to menopausal changes.

A family history such as a mother or sister with osteoporosis is associated with a higher risk of developing it herself. Other factors that might give her a higher risk are:

• an established menopause before the age of 45 years
• being underweight
• smoking
• taking little physical exercise
• treatment with corticosteroids

- a poor diet with little calcium or vitamin D intake
- excess alcohol intake
- a fragility fracture (one occurring with minimal trauma such as slipping over)
- having a medical condition such as rheumatoid arthritis, malabsorption syndromes (Crohn's disease, ulcerative colitis, gluten sensitivity), liver or parathyroid disease.

Reasons for hormonal blood test

Many women ask if they can have a blood test to determine whether they are 'on the change'. If she has already stopped having periods, there is little point unless she requires investigation because of her young age. The variable level of hormones in people having periods makes hormonal blood tests largely irrelevant too (*see* Box 9.2). The only indication for blood tests is if the history is suggestive of a condition other than a straightforward menopausal transition.

Box 9.2:   Blood tests for menopausal symptoms

Follicle stimulating hormone (FSH) is only helpful if the level is in the menopausal range (over 30 IU/l). The level fluctuates widely when a woman is still having menstrual loss and is going through the perimenopause. The level is controlled by the pulsatile release of GnRH from the hypothalamus, and is affected by feedback from oestrogen and progesterone levels as well as by inhibin. Several measurements over a period of time may be required if a premature menopause is suspected.

Oestradiol levels are not useful in the diagnosis of the menopause, either premature or at the usual time, because of the variation in levels from day to day and even at various times of day. Oestradiol levels can be used to check the levels of circulating hormone before replacement of subcutaneous implants of oestrogen, or to check levels absorbed from the skin or mucus membranes. Oestrogen given orally is mainly converted to oestrone so that oestradiol levels are not helpful.

Thyroid function tests may be useful when doubt arises as to whether symptoms are actually menopausal. Tiredness, weight gain, hair loss and flushes may indicate an underactive thyroid rather than ovarian failure.

What she may know about the menopause

She may say that she has read lots about it and has just come to you for hormone replacement therapy (HRT). It is still worth establishing what she can do herself to combat the effects of the menopause.[6] She may need advice on:

- identifying the things that trigger the flushes, e.g. hot drinks, caffeine, spicy food, alcohol, and reducing or avoiding them
- wearing layers of clothing so that some can be removed easily when she has a flush
- relaxation techniques to avoid feeling stressed and rushed as anxiety can make flushes more frequent
- complementary therapy (e.g. acupuncture, homeopathy), which may also help reduce symptoms
- taking regular exercise, eating healthily and avoiding smoking
- using lubricants to make sexual intercourse more comfortable
- using plant substances that have similar effects to those of oestrogens.[7] There is some evidence that phytoestrogens may be helpful. The two important groups of foods containing phytoestrogens are: isoflavones that are found in soybeans, chick peas, red clover and probably other legumes; and lignans that are found in linseeds and smaller amounts in cereal bran, vegetables, legumes and fruit.

Be cautious about the claims for other herbal treatments, some of which may interact with prescribed medications (e.g. warfarin, antidepressants). Others may contain toxic chemicals such as pesticides, mercury, arsenic and lead. Black cohosh has been approved in Germany for treatment of the menopause, and St John's Wort can help with mild depressive symptoms.

Progesterone cream is sold for treatment of menopausal symptoms. Insufficient is absorbed to be bone-protective, or to provide protection for the endometrium if oestrogen replacement therapy is used, but women often report lessening of symptom severity.

Advising on hormone replacement therapy

If you have had a long consultation already, you might at this stage give the woman some information on HRT to take away with her. You might lend her a book[8] or video and give her some leaflets from your patient resources. Ensure that the information is as up to date as you can find because of the rapidly changing information available. She can return to see you better informed and better able to discuss the advantages and disadvantages of treatment.

If she is already well informed and the consultation has been short you might continue. Take a history for conditions that might be affected by HRT (*see* Table 9.1). Physical examination should include measurement of her blood pressure and body mass index. The Committee for Safety of Medicines (CSM) advises that clinical examination of the breasts and pelvis is not necessary

Table 9.1:   HRT and pre-existing conditions (derived from *Management of the Menopause*[9])

Condition	Effect
Asthma	Small increased risk; no worsening of pre-existing disease
Breast cancer	Vaginal oestrogens not CI; trials in progress
Cardiovascular disease	HRT not indicated for prevention. Some preparations may have favourable effects on lipids and cell oxygenation but thrombosis risk is increased. Risk/benefit calculation required on an individual basis
Cervical cancer or dysplasia	Not CI
Crohn's disease or coeliac disease	Increased risk of osteoporosis, use transdermal route to maximise absorption
Diabetes mellitus	Increased risk of osteoporosis, but also increased risk of cardiovascular disease. Risk/benefit calculation required on an individual basis
Endometrial cancer	Not CI, continuous combined is protective
Endometriosis	Small risk of reactivation but evidence poor. Continuous combined would be best choice
Epilepsy	Not CI. Phenytoin and carbamazepine users have higher risk of osteoporosis and may need higher dose because of liver enzyme induction
Fibroids	Small risk of enlargement, but evidence poor. Use continuous combined
Gall bladder disease	Increased risk of acceleration of incipient gall bladder disease (i.e. if she was going to get it, it will arrive sooner rather than later)
Hyperlipidaemia	Not CI, choose route and preparation to improve lipid profile
Hypertension	Not CI, no evidence of worsening of control when started on HRT
Liver disease	Transdermal route preferred, take specialist advice if more than mildly affected
Malignant melanoma	Epidemiological studies have not shown any association with outcome
Migraine	Not CI; transdermal route and continuous combined preferable to give smaller hormonal fluctuations
Otosclerosis	Take specialist advice, but no evidence of harm
Ovarian cancer	Take specialist advice but often not CI
Parkinson's disease	Not CI; some evidence of preventive effect
Post-transplant	Consider as option for osteoporosis prevention
Renal failure	Consider as option for osteoporosis prevention; risk of early menopause

continued opposite

Table 9.1: *continued*

Condition	Effect
Rheumatoid arthritis	Consider as option for osteoporosis prevention; no increase in disease
Systemic lupus erythematosis	Consider as option for osteoporosis prevention; no increase in disease, but remember the increased risk of thrombosis
Thyroid disease	Consider as option for osteoporosis prevention; not CI
Valvular heart disease	Not CI but consider the risk of thrombosis
Venous thrombosis	Vaginal oestrogens not CI

CI = contraindicated

except when indicated clinically and participation in national screening programmes is sufficient if there are no symptoms or signs of disease. Mammography has a higher sensitivity and specificity for breast cancer than clinical examination. Women should also be encouraged to participate in the cervical screening programme.

Hormone replacement therapy consists of an oestrogen, which may be combined with a progestogen in women who have not had a hysterectomy. The hormone(s) can be absorbed by different routes: oral, transdermal, subcutaneous, intranasal and vaginal.

Women may be given an oestrogen subcutaneous implant after a total hysterectomy and bilateral oophorectomy but this method of administration can be difficult to manage (*see* Box 9.3).

Box 9.3:   Management of oestrogen implants

Use of subcutaneous implants was associated with tachyphylaxis i.e. menopausal symptoms returned and a further implant was given even while the blood levels of oestradiol were high. Very high levels of oestradiol could be attained after repeated implants. Although the risk of this occurring appeared low, some women were intolerant of symptoms and demanded early replacement of the implant. The management now advised is not to replace an implant until oestradiol levels are no higher than 400 pmol/l.[10]

Tibolone is a synthetic hormone that has mixed oestrogenic, progestogenic and androgenic actions, and is used by women who do not want to have bleeding (*see* Box 9.4)

Box 9.4: How tibolone differs from oestrogen plus progestogen replacement
therapy

- It alleviates menopausal symptoms like oestrogen, but its effect on the endometrium is like that of progestogen. Cyclical bleeding is not promoted.
- Vaginal cell maturation is normalised and symptomatic atrophic vaginitis is
  relieved with reduction in vaginal dryness and dyspareunia.
- Randomised studies have shown improvements in mood compared with
  placebo and similar effects on adverse mood to conventional HRT.
- It significantly reduces sex hormone binding globulin and has some androgenic effects. Improvements in sexual functioning are greater than those
  seen with conventional HRT.
- It has oestrogenic effects on bone density.
- Tibolone inhibits proliferation of human breast cells. The incidence of breast
  tenderness is low and breast density is not increased unlike conventional
  HRT. It is not known if this translates into clinical significance for the risk of
  breast cancer.
- No increase in thrombotic events in women taking tibolone have been reported
  in the literature (but this may be due to the small numbers of women taking it).

Tibolone does not suit every woman and may provide inadequate relief of
symptoms in some women. Some complain of progestogen-like side-effects.[11]

The minimum dose that has been shown to be protective of bone mass is
shown in Box 9.5 but lower doses may be effective in some women.

Box 9.5: Minimum bone sparing doses of HRT [9]

Oestradiol oral	1–2 mg
Oestradiol patch	25–50 µg
Oestradiol gel	1–5 g (depending on preparation)
Oestradiol implant	50 mg every six months
Conjugated equine oestrogens	0.3–0.625 mg daily

How you should start HRT

If menstruation has not stopped yet, start with a monthly (or three-monthly)
sequential cyclical preparation to try to promote a regular bleeding pattern.
Once no menstruation has occurred for 12 months, a continuous combined,
no bleed, preparation can be tried. Continuous combined preparations reduce

the endometrial cancer risk compared to sequential cyclic regimes. It is sensible to become familiar with a few of the large range of HRT therapies available and to ensure that you prescribe in a cost-effective way. Consider the cost of the preparation and the acceptability to the woman. Oral medication is generally cheaper than other delivery systems, but discuss what the woman would prefer – tablets, transdermal patches or gels, nasal spray, or vaginal ring.

Switching from sequential to continuous combined therapy

Change over when the woman is postmenopausal. At the age of 54 years, 80% of women are postmenopausal. Most women who have had six months without any bleeding, or who have had raised FSH levels after the mid-40s, are postmenopausal.

Protecting the endometrium in women who have not had a hysterectomy

Progestogens are added to reduce the risk of hyperplasia and carcinoma of the endometrium that occurs with unopposed oestrogen. Women who have had endometrial ablation need progestogens, as it cannot be assumed that all the endometrium has been removed. Standard sequential or continuous combined therapies contain suitable levels of progestogen to protect the endometrium. Consult a reference text for acceptable doses of progestogen for endometrial protection if using a non-standard preparation. Although not licensed yet in the UK for this indication, a Mirena intrauterine system can be used to provide both contraception and endometrial protection and can be particularly useful if the woman has unacceptable progestogenic side-effects such as bloating, acne or premenstrual syndrome symptoms.[12] Changing the progestogen to dydrogesterone may also reduce progestogenic side-effects. Most women who have had a hysterectomy can take oestrogen alone.

Treatment of urogenital symptoms

These are best treated with vaginally administered low dose natural oestrogens, such as oestriol by cream or pessary, or oestradiol by tablet or from a ring. Long-term treatment is needed or symptoms will recur. With the recommended dosage regimes, no endometrial effects should occur and it is not necessary to add a progestogen.

How long should HRT be continued?[9]

- *Treatment of flushes and other symptoms*: continue while symptoms affect the quality of life, but re-evaluate benefits and risks after symptoms have resolved and have a trial without HRT.
- *Prevention or treatment of osteoporosis*: HRT would have to be continued for life as bone mineral density falls once treatment is stopped. Most women and their health professionals will choose to transfer to other bone-protective agents once menopausal symptoms have stopped.
- *Premature menopause*: continue until at least the median age of menopause (51 years), then re-evaluate benefits and risks.

Breast cancer and HRT

Several studies have shown that women using combined HRT have a higher risk of breast cancer.[13–16] The risk with oestrogen-only HRT appears to be less than for combined therapy. The extra risk only becomes apparent for women who are taking HRT after the usual age of the menopause. The 'Million Women Study'[16] estimates that in the last ten years 20 000 extra cases of breast cancer in women aged 50–65 years of age may have been associated with the use of HRT. Translating this into the absolute risk of developing breast cancer in this age group, it changes the risk from 7 per 1000 to 11 per 1000.

Five years after stopping HRT, the woman's risk of breast cancer is the same as for women who have never taken it. If women are taking HRT at the time their breast cancer is diagnosed, their life expectancy does not seem to be reduced. It is not known if this is because cancers are diagnosed at an earlier stage in HRT users or because the HRT has an effect on the cancer (*see* Table 9.2).

Table 9.2: Additional breast cancers occurring over time with use of HRT[14,15]

	Length of HRT use		
	2 years	*5 years*	*10 years*
Oestrogen alone	0.7	2	5
Combined HRT	2	8	22

Thrombosis risk and HRT [9,13]

It is now clear that HRT increases the risk of thrombosis, so the risks and benefits need to be established at every review. The background risk of thrombosis in menopausal women is about 1 in 10 000 women per year.

Using HRT will increase this by about 2–4 extra women in every 10 000 developing a thrombosis each year.

Non-oestrogen treatments

After discussion about the benefits and risks of HRT you may advise against HRT or the woman may decide against it. Other medication should then be considered if she has risk factors.

Osteoporosis

If the main indication for treatment is prevention or treatment of osteoporosis then other medication may be preferable (*see* Table 9.3).

Table 9.3: Prevention and treatment of osteoporosis: Royal College of Physicians' grade of recommendations for therapy[4]

	Spine	*Hip*
Etridronate	A	B
Aledronate	A	A
Risedronate	A	A
Calcium and vitamin D	ND	A
Calcium	A	B
Calcitriol	A	ND
Calcitonin	A	B
Selective oestrogen receptor modulators (*see* Box 9.6)	A	ND

A = good evidence from randomly controlled trials.
B = evidence from observational or case controlled trials.
ND = not demonstrated.

Box 9.6: Selective oestrogen receptor modulators (SERMs)[11]

This class of compounds act as oestrogens in some locations and anti-oestrogens in others. Tamoxifen, the first SERM, is widely used as a treatment for breast cancer containing oestrogen receptors. Its use is associated with a raised risk of venous thrombosis and of endometrial cancer.

Raloxifene, the second SERM to be commercially available, has shown a good reduction of the risk of breast cancer in people receiving it for prevention of osteoporosis. The coronary heart risk was also reduced. Further long-term studies are needed to confirm these findings.

SERMs increase hot flushes and the risk of venous thrombosis. Trials are underway to determine if a combination of a low-dose oestradiol with a SERM might improve the risk profile. This would relieve hot flushes, protect the breast and bone mass and, it is hoped, have a neutral effect on the endometrium.

Hot flushes and other symptoms[17]

Try progestogens: e.g. norethisterone 5 mg/day or megestrol acetate 40 mg/day. Clonidine was shown in one trial to reduce flushing but was used transdermally and is not available in the UK in this formulation. Selective serotonin reuptake inhibitors (SSRIs) e.g. venlafaxine/paroxetine are not licensed for this indication but early results from trials suggest they may be helpful.

Vaginal atrophy

Vaginal lubricants can be used.

Women who might need referral for specialist advice[9]

Most women can be managed in primary care but some conditions may prompt specialist referral as follows:

*   *abnormal bleeding*:
    *   before starting HRT – a sudden change in menstrual pattern, intermenstrual bleeding, postcoital bleeding or a postmenopausal bleed
    *   sequential HRT – a change in the pattern of withdrawal bleed or breakthrough bleeding (BTB)
    *   continuous combined HRT – BTB for more than 4-6 months after starting or that is not lessening. Bleeding after complete amenorrhoea
*   *multiple treatment failures* after more than three types of HRT preparations tried. List what has been given and the problems encountered
*   *confirmed venous thrombosis*: either personal history or in a first-degree relative under the age of 50 years
*   *premature menopause*: to determine the reason for the menopause under 40 years of age
*   *osteoporosis risk*: to help with the assessment for treatment and response to treatment (refer for bone mineral density scans if available in your area)
*   *previous or high risk of hormone-dependent cancer*: e.g. breast, ovarian, endometrial cancer.

Collecting data to demonstrate your learning, competence, performance and standards of service delivery: the menopause

Example cycle of evidence 9.1

- Focus: clinical care
- Other relevant focus of evidence: working with colleagues

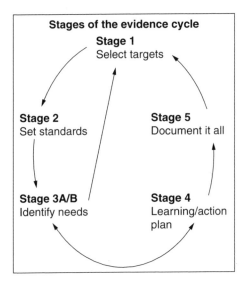

Stages of the evidence cycle

Stage 1
Select targets

Stage 2
Set standards

Stage 5
Document it all

Stage 3A/B
Identify needs

Stage 4
Learning/action plan

Box 9.7: Case study

The practice nurse refers Mrs Muddle back to you. You think you remember a discussion about her using local oestrogen, but you cannot find anything in her medical record. From her history and examination, local oestrogen would be indicated clinically. Afterwards you look again through her consultation record. By chance, you find a recent previous entry for 'urinary tract infection' and find your previous discussion there. You had sent off a midstream urine (MSU) but you had not requested her to re-attend when the result had not shown any infection. You suspect this was because of the misleading Read coding. You had not connected the negative results of the MSU with her complaints of frequency, dysuria and 'soreness down below'.

This is just an example. Keep your task simple. You could choose three or four cycles of evidence to demonstrate your competence each year.

Stage 1: Select your aspirations for good practice

The excellent GP:

- makes an adequate assessment of the patient's condition, based on the history and, if indicated, an appropriate examination
- provides or arranges investigations or treatment where necessary
- keeps clear, legible and contemporaneous records that include clinical findings, decisions made, information given to patients and any treatments given or prescribed.

Stage 2: Set the standards for your outcomes

Outcomes might include:

- the way learning is applied
- a learnt skill
- a protocol
- a strategy that is implemented
- meeting recommended standards.

- Demonstrate consistent best practice in assessment and treatment of postmenopausal urogenital atrophy.
- Demonstrate consistent best practice in keeping good patient medical records.

Stage 3A: Identify your learning needs

- Determine what barriers to best practice exist by a record review of 20 other patients who present in a similar way to Mrs Muddle (above).
- Incorporate a check to review the diagnostic coding under which information is recorded before saving the record. Use a reminder sticker or message on the computer screen to trigger the check. This is useful for other conditions when the diagnosis changes during the course of the consultation.

Stage 3B: Identify your service needs

Any of the needs assessment exercises in 3A may also reveal service needs.

- Track what happens to MSU reports when received by the practice.
- Discuss with other health professionals their response to MSU results that are reported as 'negative' or 'white blood cells and no growth' and what they record that the patient should be told.
- Discuss with practice staff what information they give to patients about their MSU results from the comments written on the report by the health professional.
- Undertake a SWOT analysis of the way records are made and kept (storage, paper based, electronic, coding etc.) with others on the practice team.

Stage 4: Make and carry out a learning and action plan

- Read about urogenital atrophy, its symptoms and treatment.
- Write up the record review (which shows perhaps that most women are being treated in accordance with best practice but that a few women with urinary symptoms of urogenital atrophy are not having a discussion of treatment options).
- Discuss the record review with other health professionals and agree to change the wording of the instructions to the practice staff from 'no infection' to 'no infection, please see the doctor if you still have symptoms' to provide a fail-safe mechanism.
- Meet with the practice staff to go through with them the reasons for the change in wording and other improvements in the way records are made and stored, because of the review and SWOT analysis.

Stage 5: Document your learning, competence, performance and standards of service delivery

- Use a reminder on the practice audit calendar and repeat the record review in six months to confirm that the changes are working.
- Document the discussion of your results with other health professionals and obtain their feedback.
- Obtain feedback from the practice manager and practice staff about interactions with patients over the giving of MSU results and record the results in your portfolio.
- Keep notes of SWOT analysis and subsequent plan.

Box 9.8: Case study continued

The fail-safe mechanism for Mrs Muddle had been a consultation with the practice nurse. Her complaints improved following the use of local oestrogen therapy. You wanted to prevent the situation of confused recording happening with other patients, so you review the situation in six months at a multidisciplinary practice meeting. The practice staff understand better the importance of follow up of negative investigations. The changes in recording the MSU results and methods of passing on the information to patients are working well. The practice staff feel, and patients and other staff confirm, that they have become more helpful in directing patients appropriately. You and other health professionals are more aware, and more proactive, about best practice in managing patients with urogenital atrophy.

Example cycle of evidence 9.2

- Focus: maintaining good medical practice
- Other relevant focus of evidence: working with colleagues

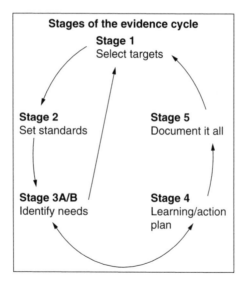

Stages of the evidence cycle

Stage 1
Select targets

Stage 2
Set standards

Stage 5
Document it all

Stage 3A/B
Identify needs

Stage 4
Learning/action plan

Box 9.9:   Case study

Mrs Manager is annoyed that the practice nurse has referred her back to the doctor because she has had irregular bleeding. She explains impatiently to you that she often manipulates the timing of her bleed, as it is more convenient to do that in her busy life. She has been taking a sequential hormone pack for seven years and is now 56 years old. She is definite that she needs to continue with HRT.

This is just an example. Keep your task simple. You could choose three or four cycles of evidence to demonstrate your competence each year.

Stage 1: Select your aspirations for good practice

The excellent GP:

- keeps his or her knowledge and skills up to date throughout their working life, through continuing educational activities that maintain and develop competence and performance
- works with colleagues to monitor and maintain the quality of care provided
- takes part in regular and systematic medical and clinical audit and makes improvements accordingly.

Stage 2: Set the standards for your outcomes

Outcomes might include:

- the way learning is applied
- a learnt skill
- a protocol
- a strategy that is implemented
- meeting recommended standards.

- Demonstrate knowledge about best practice for the provision of HRT.
- Demonstrate best practice in the management of patients requiring HRT.

Stage 3A: Identify your learning needs

- Find out best current practice in the provision of HRT especially about sequential and combined preparations and control of bleeding and compare with your own practice.
- Feedback from practice nurse colleagues about patients' comments relating to your care.

Stage 3B: Identify your service needs

> Any of the needs assessment exercises in 3A may also reveal service needs.

- Audit the use of sequential HRT in the practice including setting standards. For example you might agree that 100% of women on HRT should have had a discussion of continuous combined therapy between the ages of 52 and 54 years and anyone remaining on sequential HRT after the age of 54 years should have informed consent for that course of action recorded in their medical record.
- Discuss with relevant staff the guidelines under which the practice nurse is supervising the management of patients with menopausal problems, to determine whether any amendments are required. Determine what gaps there are in their knowledge.

Stage 4: Make and carry out a learning and action plan

- Perform a literature search for recent recommendations, especially any systematic reviews, for current best practice on HRT.
- Obtain guidelines for running a menopause clinic from an authoritative source, e.g. the British Menopause Society.[18]

Stage 5: Document your learning, competence, performance and standards of service delivery

- Incorporate and disseminate the new information in the guidelines for the menopause clinic and for the clinicians.
- Re-audit the use of sequential HRT to confirm that the changes agreed are being implemented.

Box 9.10:   Case study continued

You discuss continuous combined therapy with Mrs Manager and she is very pleased to change. She is even more pleased when you review her at three months and she has not had any bleeding at all since changing the formulation.

Example cycle of evidence 9.3

- Focus: relationships with patients
- Other relevant focus of evidence: working with colleagues

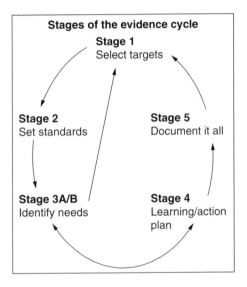

Box 9.11:   Case study continued

Mrs Manager wonders why you did not suggest a change of treatment before and you apologise – saying tactfully that she looks so young it had not crossed your mind before! You discuss Mrs Manager with the practice nurse who runs the menopause clinic with you. Both of you feel that the patient–nurse or patient–doctor interactions with this assertive woman, who was always in a hurry, had affected the quality of care that she had received.

This is just an example. Keep your task simple. You could choose three or four cycles of evidence to demonstrate your competence each year.

Stage 1: Select your aspirations for good practice

The excellent GP:

- empowers patients to take decisions about their management
- apologises appropriately when things go wrong, and has an adequate complaint procedure in place.

Stage 2: Set the standards for your outcomes

Outcomes might include:

- the way learning is applied
- a learnt skill
- a protocol
- a strategy that is implemented
- meeting recommended standards.

- Demonstrate consistent best practice in patient relationships.
- Demonstrate that you recognise when your management has not gone as well as it should, apologise appropriately to the patient and take steps to remedy the deficiency.

Stage 3A: Identify your learning needs.

- Recognise the type of doctor–patient interaction that creates barriers to best management from feedback from patients.

Stage 3B: Identify your service needs

Any of the needs assessment exercises in 3A may also reveal service needs.

- Enable colleagues, and staff for whom you are responsible, to recognise and attempt to remove the barriers to best management.
- Undertake a 360° feedback survey within the clinicians and the practice manager of the practice team, enquiring particularly about colleagues' perceived relationships with patients.
- Organise a validated patient survey (*see* page 24).

Stage 4: Make and carry out a learning and action plan

- Ask a colleague who has done assertiveness training to facilitate role play scenarios of difficult patient–staff interactions. The scenarios are to include those where the patient is very authoritative resulting in the staff member behaving in a subservient or resentful manner.
- Learn how to use that recognition of doctor–patient interaction to modify your consultation style appropriately.

Stage 5: Document your learning, competence, performance and standards of service delivery

- You and the practice nurse discuss your reflective diary records of inter-actions with other authoritative patients and record your conclusions about your improvement.
- Keep records of patient and 360° surveys and subsequent planned changes.

Box 9.12:   Case study continued

You feel that you have identified and learnt how to improve your management of powerful patients who want rapid consultations.

Example cycle of evidence 9.4

- Focus: working with colleagues
- Other relevant focus of evidence: teaching and training

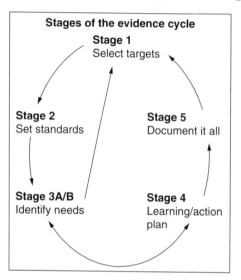

Box 9.13: Case study

Your practice nurse with whom you run the menopause clinic is going on maternity leave in four months' time. A practice in another area wants to add a menopause clinic to their sexual health provision and asks if you can advise them.

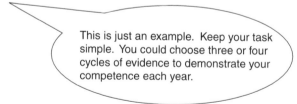

This is just an example. Keep your task simple. You could choose three or four cycles of evidence to demonstrate your competence each year.

Stage 1: Select your aspirations for good practice

The excellent GP in relationships with colleagues:

- is supportive of other team members when there are difficulties with health, conduct or performance

- has satisfactory arrangements for handing over responsibility for patients, both for communicating information and for the quality of the care they will receive, when they are not available to provide it
- makes suitable arrangements for the referral of patients to a healthcare professional of known competence or accountability to provide additional facilities or care

and in teaching and training:

- contributes to the education of students or colleagues willingly
- develops the skills, attitudes and practices of a competent teacher if he/she has responsibilities for teaching
- ensures that students and junior colleagues are properly supervised in line with responsibilities he/she has for teaching them.

Stage 2: Set the standards for your outcomes

Outcomes might include:

- the way learning is applied
- a learnt skill
- a protocol
- a strategy that is implemented
- meeting recommended standards.

- Demonstrate and communicate consistent best practice in providing clinical care for menopausal problems.
- Demonstrate and communicate consistent best practice in providing services for patients who require advice and treatment for menopausal problems.

Stage 3A: Identify your learning needs

- Assess teaching and training skills e.g. external assessment organised by a university as part of a postgraduate course.
- Review written materials for training with peer discussion to give you more insights.
- Check that the knowledge and skills you are imparting are up to date and best practice – compare against guidelines.

Stage 3B: Identify your service needs

> Any of the needs assessment exercises in 3A may also reveal service needs.

- Find out about provision for maternity leave and how the practice nurse might be supported back into being a full member of the team after her return to work. You could consult the human resources expert in the PCO.
- Discuss how the dual demands of service provision and personal health maintenance can be balanced with your mentor.
- Establish who is available to take over the practice nurse's role and what training the new person will require, by discussion with the local nurse manager.

Stage 4: Make and carry out a learning and action plan

- Attend a refresher course on teaching and training.
- Write, and obtain feedback on, training materials for the topic.
- Read widely about the subject of the menopause – literature for both GPs and patients.
- Integrate the training needs of the practice nurse's replacement with those of the staff from the other area to maximise the training opportunities.

Stage 5: Document your learning, competence, performance and standards of service delivery

- Ask for feedback from the pregnant practice nurse about whether her needs have been met.
- Log the feedback on your teaching, training and written materials.

Box 9.14:   Case study continued

The practice nurse decides to return to work part-time after her maternity leave. The practice offers her replacement a permanent contract to job share with her and to provide some extra services in the practice. Your colleagues from the other area set up a successful menopause referral clinic and you are able to interchange information and provide support for each other. The two centres join to start some research.

References

1   Bungay GT, Vessey MP and McPherson CK (1980) Study of symptoms in middle life with special reference to the menopause. *BMJ.* **281**: 181–3.

2   Nugent D and Balen A (1999) Pregnancy in the older woman. *Journal of the British Menopause Society.* **5**: 132–4.

3   Kaufert PA, Gilbert P and Tate R (1992) The Manitoba project; a re-examination of the link between depression and the menopause. *Maturitas.* **14**: 143–55.

4   Anonymous (1999) *Osteoporosis. Clinical guidelines for prevention and treatment.* Royal College of Physicians, London.

5   Black DM, Steinbuch M, Palermo L *et al.* (2001) An assessment tool for predicting fracture risk in postmenopausal women. *Osteoporos Int.* **12**: 519–28.

6   Guthrie JR (1999) Role of lifestyle approaches in the management of the menopause. *Journal of the British Menopause Society.* **5**: 25–8.

7   Ernst E (1999) Herbal remedies as a treatment of some frequent symptoms during menopause. *Journal of the British Menopause Society.* **5**: 117–20.

8   Rees M, Purdie D and Hope S (2003) *The Menopause. What you need to know.* BMS Publications, Marlow.

9   Rees M and Purdie DW (eds) (2002) *Management of the Menopause* (3e). The British Menopause Society, Marlow.

10 Buckler HM, Kalsi PK, Cantrill JA and Anderson DC (1995) An audit of oestradiol levels and implant frequency in women undergoing subcutaneous implant therapy. *Clin Endocrinol (Oxf).* **42(5)**: 445–50.

11 Davis SR (2003) Menopause: new therapies. *Menopause Journal of Australia.* **178(12)**: 634–7. Full text available with references on http://www.mja.com.au.

12 Raudaskoski T, Tapanainen J, Tomas E *et al.* (2002) Intrauterine 10 microgram and 20 microgram levonorgestrel systems in postmenopausal women receiving oral oestrogen therapy: clinical endometrial and metabolic response. *Br J Obstet Gynaecol.* **109**: 135–44.

13 Rymer J, Wilson R and Ballard K (2003) Making decisions about hormone replacement therapy. *BMJ.* **326**: 322–6.

14 Collaborative Group on Hormonal Factors in Breast Cancer (1997) Breast cancer and hormone replacement therapy: collaborative reanalysis of data from 51 epidemiological studies of 52 705 women with breast cancer and 108 411 women without breast cancer. *Lancet.* **350**: 1047–59.

15 Writing Group for the Women's Health Initiative Investigators (2002) Risks and benefits of estrogen plus progestin in healthy postmenopausal women: principal results from the Women's Health Initiative randomized controlled trial. *JAMA.* **288**: 321–33.

16 Million Women Study Collaborators (2003) Breast cancer and hormone replacement therapy in the Million Women Study. *Lancet.* **362**: 419–27.

17   Godlee F (ed.) (2003) Menopausal symptoms. *Clin Evid.* **9**: 2074–83.

18   http://www.the-bms.org.

Further reading

- Rees M and Purdie DW (eds) (2003) *Management of the Menopause* (3e). BMS Publications Ltd, Marlow. This publication contains a large number of references and suggestions for further reading on all aspects of the menopause.
- http://www.the-bms.org and *The Journal of the British Menopause Society* give information to help to keep you up to date with new information and controversies.
- http://www.menopausematters.co.uk offers practical information on the menopause and HRT, including subjects like contraception in the peri-menopause. The clinician-led site is aimed mainly at patients, but also has a section aimed at health professionals who want to keep up with their patients!

10

Teenager-friendly consultations

Box 10.1: Case study

Miss Blemish, a girl of 16 years old, attends your Monday evening surgery. She requests that you prescribe her something for her acne and casually mentions that she missed taking one of her contraceptive pills yesterday and isn't sure what to do next.

What issues you should cover

Show an interest in her skin problems. What might look like a minor condition to you might be a major cause of concern to her. Alternatively, Miss Blemish may have chosen to consult you about her acne as a first stage in asking for help with her contraception or more specifically to find out what to do about forgetting to take her contraceptive pills. You may need to positively build up her trust in you if she is fearful about any lack of privacy or confidentiality in the practice. Your good relationship may help to reinforce your medical advice and encourage her compliance with any treatments you prescribe.

Deal with the presenting condition – in this case acne

Look at the sites of the acne and record the severity of the acne in a factual way so that you can judge the extent of improvement at follow-up consultations. Sites may include the face, upper trunk and shoulders where most of the pilosebaceous follicles are situated.

Explain to Miss Blemish how acne arises so that she understands more about her condition. Tell her about the increase in keratin at the openings of the pilosebaceous ducts which together with the increase in sebum production result in the formation of open comedones (blackheads) and closed comedones (whiteheads). These are usually colonised with *Propionobacterium acnes*. Describe the subsequent inflammatory papules and pustules. In severe acne there may also be formation of nodules and scars. Let her know that the aims of treatment are to improve the look of the skin and to prevent scarring as the acne lesions heal. She should also be aware that improvement will be gradual and will take two to three months to become apparent.

Mild acne should respond to benzoyl peroxide e.g. Miss Blemish could start with a 2.5% low-strength gel applied at night. Warn her that the gel could irritate her skin and should be tried out on a small area first and not used more frequently than directed. Advise her that benzoyl peroxide may bleach clothes (or pillow cases). You can tell Miss Blemish that you will be able to increase the strength of benzoyl peroxide to 10% at two-weekly intervals if that proves necessary.[1]

If Miss Blemish has already tried benzoyl peroxide with insufficient effect or found it too much of an irritant on her skin, you may consider prescribing a topical antibiotic such as erythromycin and zinc (Zineryt). If her acne consists mainly of comedones, you may try a topical retinoid such as tretinoin or isotretinoin over several months. Increasing the dose slowly from a low strength, such as 0.025% every other night, should enable any side-effects of redness and peeling skin to settle before increasing the frequency to once or twice a day or using stronger applications. For acne that is really moderate rather than mild, you might plump for an oral antibiotic instead of a topical preparation, either alone or in combination with benzoyl peroxide or a topical retinoid. Oxytetracycline 500 mg twice daily for three months in the first instance is the usual recommended dose for oral antibiotics, changing after that time to another antibiotic if there has been no improvement, but continuing for up to two years if results are good – on the minimum dosage necessary such as 500 mg per day or even 250 mg daily.[1] You might opt for alternative antibiotics such as trimethoprim 100–200 mg twice daily, doxycycline 100 mg daily or minocycline 100 mg daily (but take care with minocycline to monitor Miss Blemish for hepatotoxicity).[1,2] Ensure that she knows that she should not take the antibiotics if there is any chance she might be pregnant or planning pregnancy; if oral antibiotics are unavoidable, erythromycin 250–500 mg twice daily is the only oral antibiotic that is not contraindicated.

Another alternative line of therapy to consider is changing her contraceptive pill to one that is less androgenic, avoiding those containing levonorgestrel or high doses of norethisterone. You might start her on Dianette (cyproterone acetate and ethinylestradiol) which is licensed for the treatment of contraception when it is being used primarily for acne. Warn Miss Blemish about the four-fold risk of thrombosis on Dianette compared to other contraceptives containing levonorgestrel and be ready to change her pill to a safer combination once her acne is under control. If Miss Blemish has severe acne (i.e. nodular and/or scarring acne) or is in real psychological distress about it, you will probably be ready to refer her to a dermatologist for oral isotretinoin. You might start treatment with Dianette or a second-line antibiotic such as minocycline with benzoyl peroxide in the morning and a topical retinoid at night, while awaiting the appointment with a dermatology specialist if there is going to be a delay of more than two weeks. A blood test for liver function and lipids will be useful to the local dermatologist if you think he or she will start Miss Blemish on oral roaccutane.

If you are seeing Miss Blemish after she has suffered a relapse in the control of her acne, her previous response to the various medications will influence her current treatment options.[3]

Advice about missed contraceptive pills[4]

Find out from Miss Blemish how many pills she has taken in this pack before the missed pill and whether this is the only one she has missed in this pack. Work through with her the rules for missed contraceptive pills, described in Box 10.2. Calculate if she has been at risk of unprotected sex in the last few days, if for instance she has not restarted the next packet of her contraceptive pills nine days after finishing her previous pack – and prescribe emergency contraception (*see* Chapter 5) if required.

Information about missed pills needs frequent repetition and reinforcement with a leaflet for all those on oral contraceptives. Emphasise the dangers of lengthening the pill-free week to more than seven days. By the end of the pill-free week follicles may only be a couple of days away from being ripe enough to release the ovum and only become quiescent on restarting the contraceptive pill. Fortunately, this degree of activity only occurs in a few women, but nearly a quarter of women show some ovarian follicular activity by the seventh pill-free day.

Discuss where Miss Blemish keeps her pills as she is living at home. If she has to conceal them from other family members (especially younger brothers) she may be more likely to forget them. Encourage her to build in reminder mechanisms such as keeping the pill packet with her clean underwear, or her toothbrush, to aid regular pill taking.

Lastly, you might discuss whether an oral contraceptive is a method that suits her lifestyle, and if a longer-term contraceptive might be preferable instead. However, progestogen-only methods (an injection or implant) may worsen her tendency to acne. If she has repeated missed pills you might consider the contraceptive patch despite its higher cost. Miss Blemish might find it easier to remember to put a patch on every week – but she might find this just as difficult unless contraception is important to her. She needs to be aware of how likely pregnancy is if she is unprotected.

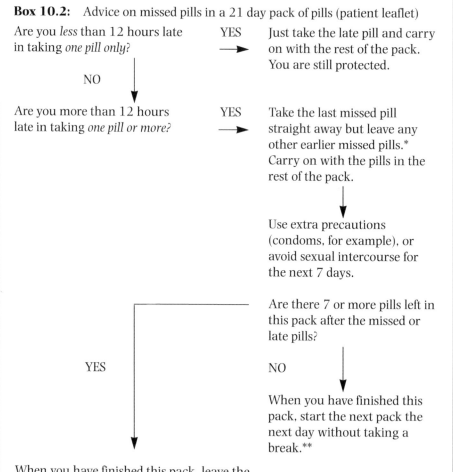

Box 10.2:   Advice on missed pills in a 21 day pack of pills (patient leaflet)

Are you *less* than 12 hours late in taking *one pill only?*   **YES** → Just take the late pill and carry on with the rest of the pack. You are still protected.

NO

Are you more than 12 hours late in taking *one pill or more?*   **YES** → Take the last missed pill straight away but leave any other earlier missed pills.* Carry on with the pills in the rest of the pack.

Use extra precautions (condoms, for example), or avoid sexual intercourse for the next 7 days.

Are there 7 or more pills left in this pack after the missed or late pills?

YES   **NO**

When you have finished this pack, start the next pack the next day without taking a break.**

When you have finished this pack, leave the usual 7 day break before starting the next pack.

*If you missed pills in the first seven days of your pack, or you have missed four or more after you have taken the first seven pills, you may need emergency contraception *as well*. Talk to a nurse or doctor.

**If you are on a 28 day pack, you must identify the inactive pills and discard them in the calculations above. Speak to a doctor or nurse for advice.

Encouraging young people to adopt a healthy lifestyle

It may be a good time to check with Miss Blemish if she smokes cigarettes, while you are reviewing her safety on the contraceptive pill. Oral contraceptives have been shown to have an adverse effect on deaths from ischaemic heart disease only in women who were currently smoking 15 or more cigarettes per day.[5]

Remind her that using condoms routinely gives her added safety against pregnancy, if she does forget future pills, and from sexually transmitted infections. Rates of sexually transmitted infections as a consequence of not using a barrier method of contraception are soaring in young people – *see* Chapter 5.

We know the range of clinical conditions that usually bring young people to the GP. Conditions leading to consultations with GPs in one study of 700 young people in the West Midlands are listed in Table 10.1.[6,7] Teenagers may well consult you with a dermatological condition such as acne, but have an underlying mental health problem which they conceal or of which they are unaware. It is startling how few young people consulted their GPs with a psychological condition or other mental health problem in this study and it is likely that this finding is generalisable to elsewhere in the UK.

Table 10.1: Reasons for consultation with a GP, over a 12 month period (total number = 700 young people)[6]

Condition	Number per hundred
Respiratory conditions	35
Dermatological conditions	28
Musculoskeletal conditions	22
Otorhinological conditions	18
Urogenital conditions	9
Gastrointestinal conditions	8
Psychological conditions	4
Ophthalmic conditions	4
Miscellaneous conditions	14

Teenagers like Miss Blemish tend to present lots of health queries if encouraged by the interest of their GP or practice nurse. Table 10.2 describes how frequently young people consulted health professionals and others for common conditions. Teenagers are most likely to go to their GP for skin complaints and least likely to go to the GP in respect of smoking or STIs. The very high numbers of young people not using any source of advice from a health professional is a serious cause of concern.[7,8]

In this study, the GP seems to be regarded as a useful source of help for diet. Use the opportunity to promote sensible eating and warn against the dangers of anorexia nervosa.

Another important feature of a healthy lifestyle is limiting alcohol. Although Miss Blemish is only 16 years old, she is likely to be drinking alcohol. Statistics tell us that just over half (53%) of 15–16-year-old girls and 58% of boys of the same age will have had so much alcohol as to be 'really drunk' on at least two

Table 10.2: Types of people consulted for different health conditions by 15–16 year olds[8]

Condition	Percentages of professionals or others consulted for specific conditions				
	No one	GP	School nurse	Clinic staff	Other
Spots/acne	39	51	1	5	4
Diet	50	31	9	4	7
Smoking	64	16	9	3	8
Pregnancy	34	25	4	30	5
STIs	58	18	9	8	6

occasions. Fifteen per cent of girls and 21% of boys will have done so on more than ten occasions.[9,10] Other surveys have corroborated these findings. Drinking alcohol at parties and friends' houses is a normal part of the social life of a teenager. Drinking alcohol increases the likelihood of having sex, and reduces the likelihood of using contraception. One survey of 16–19 year olds found that 19% reported that, after drinking alcohol, they had had sex which they had later regretted, and 10% said they had had unsafe sex after drinking alcohol.[11]

Providing teenager-friendly services

You need to look at all aspects of the way you provide your services for Miss Blemish and her peers. Look at the information they have when they are considering making an appointment at the practice, what flexibility exists in booking a consultation, especially in an emergency, and the welcoming atmosphere of the waiting room and staff. Consider the ways in which the practice team involves teenagers in making decisions about options for treatment and the resources you have for sharing information about health matters. Look at staff communication skills with young people and how arrangements for follow up are made.

A study of communication with teenagers in general practice found that they wanted:

- flexible, non-embarrassing access to non-judgemental healthcare
- time to explore reasons for attending within the primary care consultation
- information not lectures
- explanations in plain English and not medical jargon
- to be treated with the same respect as adults
- to be made aware of their choices in healthcare
- to be made aware of the duties of doctors and the rights of patients e.g. confidentiality.[12]

The study revealed a conflict between what GPs and teenagers viewed as being 'good' communication. GPs judged good communication as being the teenager listening to the GP, taking advice, being passive and not causing trouble. Teenagers thought good communication was being given time to explain their problems in their own way, having their health problems explained to them in language they understand and being made to feel legitimate patients. Young people studied did not believe promises of confidentiality made by health professionals, citing their collective experiences of breaches in confidentiality.[12]

Box 10.3:   Tips for providing services to teenagers[13,14]

- Discuss the practice guidelines on confidentiality with all young people (*see* Chapter 3) and make it a priority issue in the practice.
- Always offer the young person the option of being seen alone.
- Follow up young people more frequently initially to build up their trust and confidence and answer their questions and concerns.
- Only consider undertaking a pelvic examination in a young woman if pathology is expected and do not do one as a routine.
- Know the local procedures for child protection in case you find out that a young person is at risk of suffering or significant harm.
- Know and follow the Fraser recommendations for advice and prescription for the under-16 year old (*see* Chapter 3).
- Work closely with school nurses as part of the integrated provision of health advice and contraceptive services in your district.
- Provide an easily accessible help service that young people can contact for advice that they trust. This might be provided by the practice nurse or school nurse as an alternative to face-to-face consultations. You could advertise an electronic resource to offer answers to common queries about sex and other health issues. You could provide a link from your practice website (e.g. for Connexions).[15]
- Organise your practice team to look at ways to promote the teenager friendliness of the practice. Ask teenagers themselves for their views about what works.
- Identify the characteristics of the 10–18 year olds in your practice so you can plan to address their needs, boys as well as girls.
- Train GPs, nurses and receptionists about contraception as appropriate – all have their role to play in their interaction with teenagers coming in for contraception.
- Inform young people as to what the practice provides by posters, a practice information booklet for teenagers, and a 'birthday' letter to all young people on your list when they become 16 years old (or earlier).
- Advertise services that are available for young people outside the practice.
- Consider organising a young person's clinic run at convenient times for teenagers.
- Involve parents in the provision of services for young people and in compiling information for parents about teenagers' health.
- Offer advice and support for teenagers who do get pregnant providing information about, and referral to, supporting agencies.

How you can make an impact on young people's risk-taking behaviour

Concentrate on controlling the most common sources of risk in primary care. These include poor continuity of care, communication difficulties and informing virgins about emergency contraception. Work with teachers and parents to give them accurate information about contraception that they in turn can relay to young people. Provide information to debunk common myths that tempt young people to take unnecessary risks.

Focus on health promotion messages about safe sex whenever a young person comes for emergency contraception – safe from pregnancy, safe from infection and safe from coercion. Establish a good rapport in the emergency situation and the young person will return for more routine care when you can discuss health risks associated with smoking, excessive alcohol and substance misuse too. Tell young people more about the subsequent effects of sexual infection such as the increased rates of infertility from infection with chlamydia and the association of alcohol and drug misuse with unwanted pregnancy. Learn more about how to motivate teenagers to resist or reduce risky behaviour.

Make sure that your health promotion literature is reproduced in all the languages of your patient population. For instance, the manufacturers of the progesterone depot injection produce patient information leaflets in English, Greek, Bengali, Hindi, Chinese, Punjabi, Urdu, Gujarati and Turkish languages.

Collecting data to demonstrate your learning, competence, performance and standards of service delivery: teenager-friendly consultations

Example cycle of evidence 10.1

- Focus: clinical care
- Other relevant focus of evidence: relationships with patients

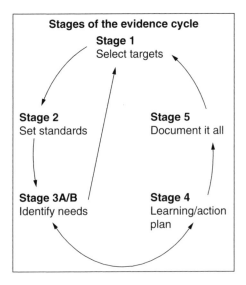

Stages of the evidence cycle

Stage 1
Select targets

Stage 2
Set standards

Stage 5
Document it all

Stage 3A/B
Identify needs

Stage 4
Learning/action plan

Box 10.4: Case study

Diana Spot has been consulting you about her acne off and on for 12 months. She is back to see you with a flare up about which she is very self-conscious. She demands that you prescribe oral roaccutane instead of benzoyl peroxide gel, as one of her friends has had this treatment with success. You look closely at the acne on her back and face to see that it is mild with some inflammation but no evidence of scarring.

This is just an example. Keep your task simple. You could choose three or four cycles of evidence to demonstrate your competence each year.

Stage 1: Select your aspirations for good practice

The excellent GP:

*   only prescribes treatments that make an effective contribution to the patient's overall management
*   is up to date with developments in clinical practice and regularly reviews his/her knowledge and performance.

Stage 2: Set the standards for your outcomes

Outcomes might include:

*   the way learning is applied
*   a learnt skill
*   a protocol
*   a strategy that is implemented
*   meeting recommended standards.

*   Demonstrate consistent best practice in prescribing acne treatments to teenagers and making referrals to a GP with special interest in dermatology or to a consultant dermatologist.

Stage 3A: Identify your learning needs

*   Ask the local pharmacist for feedback about what teenagers say about you when they come to obtain medication for acne over the counter or on prescription.
*   Capture in your reflective diary trends or young people's comments relating to problems or issues of skin conditions including acne.
*   Self-assess and reflect on your own learning needs in respect of prescribing a range of drugs for acne and their safety profiles.

Stage 3B: Identify your service needs

> Any of the needs assessment exercises in 3A may also reveal service needs.

- Undertake a teenage patient survey: consecutive teenage patients who present at the reception desk could complete a brief question sheet about the ease of making an appointment and their views on the teenager friendliness of the practice.
- Audit medication for acne as acute and repeat prescriptions by all GPs in the practice.

Stage 4: Make and carry out a learning and action plan

- Read up on the best practice in the management of acne and identify any local or national guidelines.
- Prepare for and run a teaching session about acne for medical students assigned to your practice.
- Attend an interactive workshop at a dermatology update day. Network with others with a special interest or expertise in skin conditions.
- Reflect on the presentations and cases discussed at the workshop afterwards. Draw up an action plan for the next GP partnership meeting, reflecting on the results of the audit.

Stage 5: Document your learning, competence, performance and standards of service delivery

- Re-audit after the practice has agreed changes to the initial and continuing management of acne with medication.
- Repeat the teenage patient survey after changes have been made to meet the challenges produced by the original survey.
- Repeat the collection of feedback from pharmacist.
- Repeat the recording of comments from teenagers in your reflective diary.

Box 10.5: Case study continued

You avoid commenting that Diana Spot has mild acne, but show her some pictures of various types of acne in a dermatology book so that she can gain a sense of proportion for herself. You involve her in decision making about the type of treatment she might try next. You gain her acceptance that it may take several months of treatment before there is an optimal response and that the treatment should be continued until no new lesions develop. You agree that she will give topical isotretinoin a try. She leaves, knowing that some redness and scaling of her skin may occur initially but that if she persists this should settle in time.

Example cycle of evidence 10.2

- Focus: working with colleagues
- Other relevant foci of evidence: relationships with patients; teaching and training

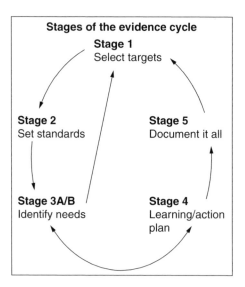

Stages of the evidence cycle

Stage 1
Select targets

Stage 2
Set standards

Stage 5
Document it all

Stage 3A/B
Identify needs

Stage 4
Learning/action plan

Box 10.6: Case study

You are the education lead in your practice team and are responsible for organising quarterly in-house learning events. The team suggested that you focus on healthcare for teenagers at the next practice team workshop.

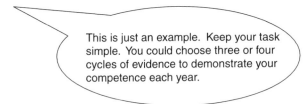

This is just an example. Keep your task simple. You could choose three or four cycles of evidence to demonstrate your competence each year.

Stage 1: Select your aspirations for good practice

The excellent GP:

- understands the health needs of the local teenage population and tries to ensure that the primary care team has skills to meet those needs.

Stage 2: Set the standards for your outcomes

Outcomes might include:

- the way learning is applied
- a learnt skill
- a protocol
- a strategy that is implemented
- meeting recommended standards.

- Create a profile of the health needs of the teenagers registered with the practice.
- Carry out an assessment of the learning needs of all members of the primary care team about the provision of healthcare for teenagers.

Stage 3A: Identify your learning needs

- Find out the statistics about mental and physical morbidity, teenage pregnancy or sexually transmitted infections from national and local public health sources and compare it with what is known from your own practice data.
- Review the records of 20 or more teenagers opportunistically or from a systematic sample. Compare the reasons for consultation with those given in the young people's survey in Table 10.1. You could also compare the treatment provided to the teenagers in your survey against best practice.
- Consider if you know how to carry out a learning needs assessment of others in the practice team. Obtain their views afterwards about your approach.

Stage 3B: Identify your service needs

> Any of the needs assessment exercises in 3A may also reveal service needs.

* Arrange for all relevant members of the practice team to self-assess their learning and training needs. Compare this with their job descriptions and with the skills needed for the services you do provide or aim to provide in the near future.
* Use a semi-structured short questionnaire to ask clinicians from local pharmacies, family planning clinics, or youth workers at youth clubs about their perceptions of your services. Include questions about the choice of staff, availability and accessibility of female or male doctors or nurses, the timing and convenience of services, and whether they receive comments about the atmosphere at the surgery.
* Use the survey of the views of young people to identify gaps across all your services.

Stage 4: Make and carry out a learning and action plan

* Update, or write, clinical protocols for teenagers who have asthma or diabetes. Look up best practice in prescribing, patient choice, and the legal aspects of consent and confidentiality. This might include reading and reflection, searching the literature or reading a review in a peer-reviewed journal, downloading a recommended protocol by a nationally recognised organisation, or a discussion with peers at a topic-based group.
* Obtain public health data about the morbidity of the teenage population and discuss it with colleagues at practice meetings or in a special interest group of the PCO.
* Plan the in-house learning event around the information you have gathered in Stage 3 and the updated clinical protocols that have been customised for the special needs of teenagers.

Stage 5: Document your learning, competence, performance and standards of service delivery

* Audit the adherence to the updated practice protocols.
* Keep the programme for the in-house learning event and the subsequent action plan for the practice.
* Keep the completed learning needs analysis of the relevant staff with their corresponding learning plans.

- Keep the health profile of the teenage practice population with information from as many sources as possible.

Box 10.7:   Case study continued

After your in-house training event, a few people volunteer to find out more from teenagers about their needs and preferences in the way you provide healthcare. You agree to start with teenagers who have asthma or diabetes.

Example cycle of evidence 10.3

- Focus: teaching and training
- Other relevant focus of evidence: confidentiality

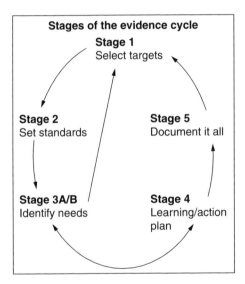

Stages of the evidence cycle
Stage 1 — Select targets
Stage 2 — Set standards
Stage 3A/B — Identify needs
Stage 4 — Learning/action plan
Stage 5 — Document it all

Box 10.8:   Case study

Laura Fear asked about whether details of her consultation really were confidential in view of the fact that her father is a caretaker in the practice. She said she was unsure about consulting you, her GP, about her contraception, and was considering visiting the local family planning clinic instead as she knows they welcome 15 year olds like herself. She has come to see you about her asthma but takes the opportunity to ask about possible side-effects of her contraception.

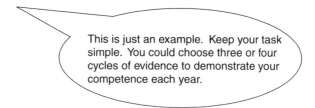

This is just an example. Keep your task simple. You could choose three or four cycles of evidence to demonstrate your competence each year.

Stage 1: Select your aspirations for good practice

The excellent GP:

- has a personal commitment to teaching and learning
- keeps patients' information confidential – including maintaining privacy to make sure that confidential information is not overheard.

Stage 2: Set the standards for your outcomes

Outcomes might include:

- the way learning is applied
- a learnt skill
- a protocol
- a strategy that is implemented
- meeting recommended standards.

- Ensure that all members of the practice team, including you, new members of staff, students or doctors in training, are familiar with guidelines for confidentiality in relation to young people receiving healthcare.

Stage 3A: Identify your learning needs

- Self-assess your knowledge and check that of team members about the guidelines for confidentiality for providing under-16 year olds with contraception or referring for termination of pregnancy.
- Plan an in-house training session on maintaining confidentiality for teenagers of different ages. Ask the opinion of an expert tutor about the method of teaching that will best convey the main messages and lead to change where necessary.

Stage 3B: Identify your service needs

> Any of the needs assessment exercises in 3A may also reveal service needs.

- Compare the practice protocol for confidentiality with the guidelines in the *Confidentiality and Young People* toolkit.[16]
- Review the induction programme for new members of staff, students on placement and doctors in training to assess the extent to which knowledge of confidentiality features.

Stage 4: Make and carry out a learning and action plan

- Find out how to establish the learning needs in an interactive multidisciplinary group from books or from a tutor.[17,18]
- Prepare for and run an interactive session on confidentiality with a special focus on teenagers. Invite others in the practice team, students, family planning or school nurses, local pharmacists, GP registrars, etc. You might use the *Confidentiality and Young People* toolkit to stimulate discussion.[16]

Stage 5: Document your learning, competence, performance and standards of service delivery

- Give a quiz to be completed by those attending the interactive session comparing their answers before and afterwards.
- Record any reported or perceived breaches of confidentiality by anyone working in the practice and how this could be avoided in future.
- Develop personal learning plans for new staff or doctors in training by the end of the induction period.

Box 10.9: Case study continued

Miss Fear is reassured by your promise not to talk to her father about her consultation. You tell her that you would expect none of the staff to mention that she has been to see you at all – now or in the future. You explain about the password system (and double-check it yourself) that ensures that there is no way that your receptionists or the caretaker can access the clinical records held on the computer. You ask the practice manager to check that everyone has attended the in-house training on confidentiality.

Example cycle of evidence 10.4

- Focus: management

GPs are required to complete the section on management in their appraisal paperwork, in relation to any responsibility they have for management outside the practice. GPs might wish to include such responsibilities within their practice role or where management responsibilities cross the interface between practice and PCO.

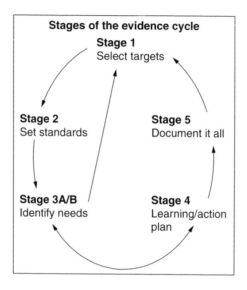

Stages of the evidence cycle

Stage 1
Select targets

Stage 2
Set standards

Stage 5
Document it all

Stage 3A/B
Identify needs

Stage 4
Learning/action plan

Box 10.10: Case study

You are the lead health professional in your practice team for sexual health. Your PCO has called upon you to represent your practice and work with other practice leads to reconfigure contraceptive services in your practice so that they are appropriate for the needs of young people.

This is just an example. Keep your task simple. You could choose three or four cycles of evidence to demonstrate your competence each year.

Stage 1: Select your aspirations for good practice

The excellent GP:

- strives to address the health priorities of his/her patient population in collaboration with the PCO – in relation to teenage contraception.

Stage 2: Set the standards for your outcomes

Outcomes might include:

- the way learning is applied
- a learnt skill
- a protocol
- a strategy that is implemented
- meeting recommended standards.

- Reconfigure contraceptive services in the practice to provide them in ways appropriate for the needs and preferences of young people.

Stage 3A: Identify your learning needs

- Self-assess your knowledge of which characteristics of young people put them most at risk of unplanned teenage pregnancy. Include assessment of knowledge about trends in sexual activity and the use of contraceptives during the teen years.
- Get recent statistics of the conception rates for your practice area from the local public health lead. Compare them with the practice data about live births and termination rates.

Stage 3B: Identify your service needs

Any of the needs assessment exercises in 3A may also reveal service needs.

- Run a search to find out how prescribing rates of contraceptives differ for teenagers living in various geographical areas of the practice.
- Compare your practice organisation with examples of good practice for making the practice teenager friendly.
- Organise, design and give out a short quiz to all young people coming to the reception desk about what would make them feel welcome and respected in healthcare settings and your practice in particular.

- Conduct a significant event audit around three consecutive cases of young people presenting as pregnant. Look at the duration of the pregnancy before consulting for the first time, the age of the teenager, whether the pregnancy was planned, whether contraception had been used previously and the reasons for the failure or non-use of contraception.

Stage 4: Make and carry out a learning and action plan

- Attend a workshop run by a teenage pregnancy lead to learn about local initiatives and meet others from local authority agencies concerned with teenage health problems.
- Read a book about the provision of contraception to teenagers and reflect on the changes needed to your current management.[4]
- Represent the practice at a workshop with the public health lead for your PCO and other practice representatives. Help to formulate changes to the way contraceptive services are provided for young people in the local area to meet local needs and preferences.

Stage 5: Document your learning, competence, performance and standards of service delivery

- Keep a record of the statistics for conception rates of teenagers in your own practice and across the PCO.
- Write a report of the changes to contraceptive service provision in the practice and changes in the numbers of patients seen.
- Collect feedback from teenagers obtaining contraception. This could be obtained by asking them to complete feedback questions slips or from notes of their responses to standard enquiries made by the GP or nurse.

Box 10.11:   Case study continued

Armed with all the information you have gathered, you are able to make a good case for the changes you feel are required in the provision of sexual health services.

References

1   Joint Formulary Committee (2003) *British National Formulary.* British Medical Association and the Royal Pharmaceutical Society of Great Britain, London.

2   Leyden JJ (1997) Therapy for acne vulgaris. *New Eng J Med.* **336**: 1156–62.

3 Chu A, Darvay A, Forsyth A *et al.* (2003) The management of the relapse of severe acne. *Guidelines.* **20**: 381.

4 Chambers R, Wakley G and Chambers S (2000) *Tackling Teenage Pregnancy: sex, culture and needs.* Radcliffe Medical Press, Oxford.

5 Vessey M, Painter R and Yeates D (2003) Mortality in relation to oral contraceptive use and cigarette smoking. *Lancet.* **362**: 185–91.

6 Jacobson L, Mellanby AR, Donovan C *et al.* (2000) Teenagers' views on general practice consultations and other medical advice. *Fam Pract.* **17**: 156–8.

7 Coleman J and Schofield J (2003) *Key Data on Adolescents.* Trust for the Study of Adolescence, TSA Publishing Ltd, Brighton.

8 Churchill R, Allen J, Denman S *et al.* (2000) Do the attitudes and beliefs of young teenagers towards general practice influence actual consultation behaviour? *Br J Gen Pract.* **50**: 953–7.

9 Hasden L, Angle H and Hickman M (1999) *Young People and Health: health behaviour in school-aged children. A report of 1997 findings.* Health Education Authority, London.

10 Eborall C and Garmeson K (2000) *Research to Inform the National Media Campaign.* Teenage Pregnancy Unit, Department of Health, London.

11 MORI (1999) *Risk Taking Among Young People.* Presentation of qualitative research to Department of Health. Cited in: C Eborall and K Garmeson (2000) *Research to Inform the National Media Campaign.* Teenage Pregnancy Unit, Department of Health, London.

12 Donovan C, Richardson G, Parry-Langdon N and Jacobson L (2001) *Bridging the Gap.* Bro Taf Health Authority, South Wales.

13 MacPherson A, Donovan C and Macfarlane A (2002) *Healthcare of Young People. Promotion in primary care.* Radcliffe Medical Press, Oxford.

14 Cooper P, Diamond I, High S and Pearson S (1994) A comparison of family planning provision: general practice and family planning clinics. *Br J Fam Plan.* **19**: 263–9.

15 www.connexions.gov.uk.

16 Donovan C (ed.) (2000) *Confidentiality and Young People. A toolkit for general practice, primary care groups and trusts.* Royal College of General Practitioners and Brook, London.

17 Chambers R, Wakley G, Iqbal Z and Field S (2002) *Prescription for Learning.* Radcliffe Medical Press, Oxford.

18 Mohanna K, Wall D and Chambers R (2003) *Teaching Made Easy* (2e). Radcliffe Medical Press, Oxford.

And finally

We hope that you have found that the stages in our 'cycle of evidence' are a useful approach to gathering information about what you need to learn. You can also use it to identify improvements you or others need to make to the way you deliver services.

It is easy to feel overwhelmed by the magnitude of the task to demonstrate that you are competent and perform consistently well as a doctor, in order to retain your licence to practise. Remember that you should be producing evidence about the breadth of your practice every five years. Take your time and select three or four cycles of evidence each year that span several headings of *Good Medical Practice* at one time.

Ask others for help. Your practice manager or the receptionists should be able to help you to collect information about what you need to learn, or about gaps in services. You can delegate much of the administrative side. Your colleagues or your patients will be well placed to help you to set your aspirations for good practice and set achievable standards for your outcomes – of learning and improvements in service delivery. Perhaps your CPD tutor can help you to develop learning and action in your PDP. These cycles of evidence will be the nucleus of your PDP. Colleagues in the team can support you in documenting the evidence of your competence, performance and subsequent standards of service delivery. Other books in this series might help you to look at specific clinical areas, especially those where quality frameworks or special interests require your attention. Remember to visit this book's supporting website, which includes useful website links: http://health.mattersonline.net.

So the evidence will be there ready to submit for appraisal interviews or revalidation, but the results will show what a good doctor you really are. This should give you increasing confidence and self-respect. Enjoy your professional glow.

Index